Feed Your Child Well

Therese Dunne, BSc Human Nutrition & Dietetics, M.I.N.D.I., currently practices as a senior paediatric diabetes dietitian at University Hospital Limerick, where she has worked since 2013. She previously practised as a senior paediatric dietitian at the Children's University Hospital Temple Street, Dublin, for thirteen years. She graduated from Trinity College Dublin and the Dublin Institute of Technology in 1998 and worked in the UK for eighteen months before joining the Dietetic Department in Temple Street. Therese provides consultations to all the children and young people attending the Paediatric Diabetes Department in University Hospital Limerick and lectures to health professionals and members of the public on aspects of paediatric nutrition. She is frequently contacted by GPs and public health nurses for nutritional advice. Therese lives in County Kerry with her husband and son.

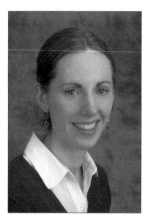

Phyllis Farrell, BSc Human Nutrition & Dietetics, M.I.N.D.I., practiced as a senior paediatric dietitian at the Children's University Hospital Temple Street, Dublin, for seven years. She graduated from Trinity College Dublin and the Dublin Institute of Technology in 1996. Originally from County Tipperary, she spent eleven years working within paediatric units and hospitals in both Ireland and the UK. She lectured to community dietitians working with children and was frequently contacted by public health nurses and GPs for nutritional advice for children. Phyllis provided consultation to several hundred children each year at Temple Street. She is now living overseas and has an interest in the area of diabetes.

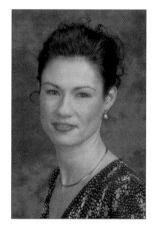

Valerie Kelly, BSc Human Nutrition & Dietetics, M.I.N.D.I., currently practices as a senior paediatric dietitian in the Children's University Hospital, Temple Street, Dublin. She graduated from Trinity College Dublin and the Dublin Institute of Technology in 2002 and began working in Temple Street immediately. Valerie provides consultations to several hundred children a year in Temple Street and lectures to health professionals and members of the public on aspects of paediatric nutrition. She is frequently contacted by GPs, public health nurses and the media for nutritional advice. Valerie lives in Bray, County Wicklow, with her husband and three children.

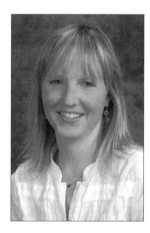

Feed Your Child Well

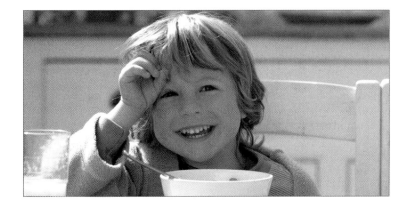

Therese Dunne

Phyllis Farrell

Valerie Kelly

THE O'BRIEN PRESS
DUBLIN

This edition first published 2017 by The O'Brien Press Ltd,
12 Terenure Road East, Rathgar, Dublin 6, D06 HD27, Ireland.
Tel: +353 1 4923333; Fax: +353 1 4922777
E-mail: books@obrien.ie
Website: www.obrien.ie
First edition published 2008, second edition published 2009, third
edition published 2011 by A. & A. Farmar Ltd.

The O'Brien Press is a member of Publishing Ireland.

ISBN: 978-1-84717-838-1

10 9 8 7 6 5 4 3 2 1
21 20 19 18 17

Printed in Drukarnia Skleniarz, Poland.
The paper used in this book is produced using pulp from managed
forests.

Published in:

DUBLIN
UNESCO
City of Literature

To all the children who come through the doors
of Temple Street Children's Hospital and especially those
we have grown to know so well.

To the little people in our lives, Nancy, Ted, Trudy & Cian.

And to the memory of Philomena Farrell, gentle loving mother
and best friend, who strongly supported the writing of this book.

Contents

Acknowledgements

There are a number of people we would like to thank in relation to the development of this book. Firstly, our wonderful colleagues and friends in Temple Street who are a great source of knowledge and support every day. We especially thank everyone in the Department of Clinical Nutrition and Dietetics: Karen Cowan, Caitriona Hensey, Lorraine Heffernan, Eimear Carroll, Fiona Ward, Marianne O'Reilly and Fiona Boyle. We would also like to thank Marie Breslin who worked in Temple Street for many years and taught us all so much.

We would also like to thank our lecturers from college, especially Mary Moloney, Sheila Sugrue, Mary Flynn, Nicky Kennedy, Paul Mathias and Mike Gibney for all their work in developing Dietetics as a qualification and encouraging us in our chosen career.

We would also like to thank our respective families for all their support and understanding during the writing of this book, especially Mike, Mark and Alan. A big thanks also to Carly Kelly and Luli Sufaj for the lovely pictures of Ross that are featured inside.

Finally we would like to extend our gratitude to Anna Farmar, our editor who worked so hard and did a wonderful job in bringing our book together. It was not easy dealing with three authors and we appreciate her understanding and patience. She was a pleasure to work with.

Therese Dunne, Phyllis Farrell and Valerie Kelly

Foreword

Dr Peter Keenan

Children engender much anxiety and sometimes bewilderment for parents. The younger they are, the more this is true. Accordingly, pre-school children and babies constitute the majority of paediatric attendances to healthcare professionals.

Gastrointestinal problems and feeding difficulties account for a large number of these attendances and the younger the infant, the more frequently problems of feeding and nutrition arise. Infants are completely dependent and are unable to give a clear history themselves. Infants and toddlers, with their rapid growth, have specific nutrition requirements and present many challenges. Poor nutritional practice, based on myth and ignorance, has massive long-term implications for the growing child.

This book has been produced by three experienced Paediatric Dietitians. It is most comprehensive, covering all aspects of child nutrition. Appropriately, there is a great emphasis on the early days and months of a child's life. There is an excellent comprehensive review of breastfeeding and transition to solid food. The layout of the text makes it very accessible with easy to understand bullet points accompanying all sections.

I would recommend this text for parents, nutritionists, nurses, midwives and medical practitioners—in short, anyone who deals with children and their nutrition. It combines solid science with practical application. I congratulate the authors and commend their efforts.

Dr PETER KEENAN
FRCPI, MRCPCH
Emergency Consultant Paediatrician
The Children's Hospital
Temple Street,
Dublin

Converting kilograms to pounds and ounces

weight conversion table

kg	lbs oz	kg	lbs oz	kg	lbs oz
3.00 kg	6 lbs 9½ oz	5.50 kg	12 lbs 1½ oz	8.0 kg	17lbs 9½ oz
3.25 kg	7 lbs 2½ oz	5.75 kg	12 lbs 10½ oz	8.25 kg	18 lbs 2½ oz
3.50 kg	7 lbs 11oz	6.00 kg	13 lbs 3 oz	8.5 kg	18 lbs 11 oz
3.75 kg	8 lbs 4oz	6.25 kg	13 lbs 12 oz	8.75 kg	19 lbs 4 oz
4.00 kg	8 lbs 13oz	6.50 kg	14 lbs 5 oz	9.0 kg	19 lbs 13oz
4.25 kg	9 lbs 6½ oz	6.75 kg	14 lbs 13½ oz	9.25 kg	20 lbs 5½ oz
4.50 kg	9 lbs 14½ oz	7.00 kg	15 lbs 6½ oz	9.5 kg	20 lbs 14½ oz
4.75 kg	10 lbs 7oz	7.25 kg	15lbs 15 oz	9.75 kg	21 lbs 7 oz
5.00 kg	11 lbs 0 oz	7.50 kg	16 lbs 8 oz	10.0 kg	22 lbs
5.25 kg	11 lbs 9 oz	7.75 kg	17 lbs 1 oz		

Understanding nutrition

1

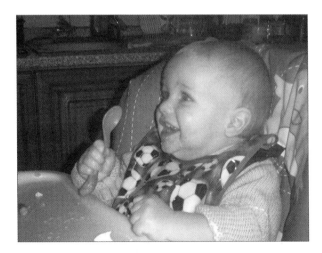

In order to grow, develop and stay healthy your child needs to eat a balanced diet which will provide enough calories for energy and essential nutrients to meet the needs of each growth stage. Energy is provided through digesting carbohydrates and fat so it is important that the diet contains sufficient quantities of these essential foods. Other essential nutrients are protein, vitamins and minerals.

Calories and energy

We all need energy in order to function—it is essential for growth, metabolism and activity. Energy is produced through digesting foods containing carbohydrate and fat. Energy in the diet is measured in units called calories, like kilowatts in light bulbs.

Because they are growing so fast babies have very high energy requirements relative to their small body size. A baby's weight will treble during the first year and length will double! While this rapid rate of growth slows down after the first year of life, toddlers still have high energy needs because of their increasing activity as well as continued growth.

During digestion carbohydrates and fat in food get broken down to release energy. During the first two years of life a high fat intake is essential to meet energy needs. Fat contains more calories than carbohydrate: 1 g of pure fat has 9 calories whereas 1 g of pure carbohydrate has only 4 calories. For this reason we refer to fat and high-fat foods as being 'energy dense'.

It is normal for the amount of calories eaten to vary from day to day and to increase during growth spurts. Babies and young children are generally good at 'sensing' how much energy their body needs.

Carbohydrates

Carbohydrate in food gets broken down during digestion to release energy. There are two main types of digestible carbohydrate in food: sugars and starches. A third type of carbohydrate is fibre which is indigestible but is very important in the diet for gut health.

Sugars

Sugars occur naturally in milk (lactose) and fruit (glucose, fructose and sucrose).

Lactose, the naturally occurring sugar in milk, is the main carbohydrate in breast milk and most formula milks. During digestion lactose is easily broken down into glucose, which provides energy to the developing brain, and galactose which is important for the development of the central nervous system. Lactose also aids the absorption of calcium and iron.

Glucose, fructose and sucrose, the three main sugars in fruit, are an integral part of the fruit and give fruit its sweet taste.

Fructose occurs naturally in many foods including honey, fruits and some root vegetables such as potatoes, parsnips and onions. Fructose is the sweetest of the naturally occurring sugars, twice as sweet as sucrose. Pure fructose can be bought in health food shops and added to foods instead of sucrose. However, just as with sucrose, eating too much fructose can cause obesity, tooth decay and other problems.

Sucrose is a combination of glucose and fructose, made from sugar beet or sugar cane. It is the sugar added to tea and coffee, sprinkled on breakfast cereals, and used in biscuits, chocolate, cakes, fizzy drinks etc. Added sugar is not necessary in the diet. It provides energy but not a single other nutrient. Calories obtained from added sugar are 'empty calories'. Too much added sugar in the diet increases the risk of tooth decay and obesity.

> **glucose** is the body's most important source of fuel and a constant supply is essential for the brain. Just as a car runs on petrol, the human body runs on glucose. It is obtainable from milk, fruit and starch.

Starch

Starch, a more complex form of carbohydrate than sugar, is found in bread, cereal, pasta, rice and grains. Starch is broken down during digestion to release glucose. As we have seen, glucose is the body's most important source of fuel and a constant supply is essential for the brain. From the age of two onwards there should be a gradual increase in the amount of energy derived from starchy foods with an equivalent decrease in energy derived from fats.

Fibre

Fibre is indigestible carbohydrate which passes through the gut bringing waste products and bacteria with it for excretion. Fibre is very important for maintaining gut health and preventing constipation. It works by trapping water in the stool to make it softer, and increasing stool weight to make it bulkier. This helps the stool move more easily and quickly through the gut.

> **fibre in the diet**
> - Traps water in the stool to make it softer.
> - Increases stool weight to make it bulkier.

There are two types of dietary fibre:
- Soluble fibre which is found in porridge or oats, beans, fruit and vegetables.
- Insoluble fibre which is found in brown bread, brown rice, vegetables and high-fibre breakfast cereals.

For good gut health both types of fibre should be included in the diet. However, too much fibre can make the diet bulky and very filling, reducing the intake of other important nutrients. Children should not fill up on high-fibre foods at the expense of more energy-rich foods.

Fibre also contains substances called phytates which, if eaten in large amounts, can interfere with the absorption of important minerals such as iron and zinc. Unprocessed bran should not be given to small children.

Fat

Fat is needed for various different functions in the body, including as a source of energy. It is a very concentrated source of energy. Fat in breast or formula milk provides half the dietary energy a baby needs. Without fat, young children would not be able to consume the volume of food necessary to provide them with enough energy to grow. Fat in children's diets should not be restricted before the age of two. By the time they are five years old they should be getting just over one third of their energy from fat. Some fats are more beneficial than others.

fat

- Provides energy and fuel for growth.
- Supplies fat-soluble vitamins A, D, E and K.
- Helps build cell membranes.
- Is important for healthy brain function.
- Protects organs such as the kidney and liver.

Healthy fats

Monounsaturated fats These fats are derived from plants such as olives, rapeseed, avocados, nuts and seeds. They are oils rather than solid fats. They do not raise cholesterol and are thought to reduce the incidence of cardiovascular disease and some cancers.

Polyunsaturated fats These are also oils rather than solid fats. They can be divided into two significant groups: omega-3 and omega-6. Omega-3 fats can come from vegetable sources such as walnut oil and flaxseed oil and are also obtained from fish oils. (See pages 10–11 for more on omega-3.) Omega-6 fats help to lower cholesterol and keep skin healthy. They are also important for a baby's brain development during pregnancy and early infancy. Arachidonic acid (AA) is the main omega-6 fatty acid. Sources include meat, eggs and dairy products. A simpler form can be found in sunflower oil, corn oil and safflower oil, nuts, seeds, whole grains and evening primrose oil.

Note Nuts should not be given to children under 5 years of age because of the danger of choking.

Less healthy fats

Saturated fats are found mainly in animal products including butter, fatty meats (especially with visible fat) and processed meats (sausage, luncheon meats). They are solid at room temperature. These fats should be eaten in moderation as they are associated with elevated risk of cardiovascular disease if eaten in excess.

Trans fat is formed when a liquid vegetable oil (unsaturated fat) is processed (hydrogenated) to form a solid fat or more stable oil that can withstand higher cooking temperatures. It is found in many products such as biscuits, cakes, crisps, chocolate and many spreads. Many fast food restaurants use partially hydrogenated oil. This fat is best avoided as much as possible.

Trans fat is not usually labelled as such on packaging. Instead look out for 'hydrogenated oil', 'partially hydrogenated oil' or 'hydrogenates' in the list of ingredients.

Trans fat
- Interferes with the action of healthy fats.
- Increases bloods levels of LDL ('bad') cholesterol.
- Lowers blood levels of HDL ('good') cholesterol.
- Increases the rate at which arteries become furred up (arteriosclerosis) increasing the risk of stroke, heart disease and cancer later in life.

Protein

Protein is essential for growth as it provides the building blocks for making new tissues such as muscle and bone. Babies require far more protein relative to their body size than children, adolescents and adults. This is because of their very rapid rate of growth.

A baby's protein requirements will be met for the first 4–6 months of life by breast milk or infant formula, taken in sufficient quantities. When solid foods are introduced during weaning protein-rich foods such as meat, fish, eggs, beans, pulses and dairy foods should be included in the diet. Small amounts of protein are also found in breads and cereals. The majority of toddlers easily meet their daily protein requirement, usually eating more than they actually need.

low-fat dairy products
Low-fat (semi-skimmed) milk or other low-fat dairy products are not recommended for children under the age of 2 years. If your child is a good eater and has a varied diet you could introduce these products after the second birthday. Skimmed milk is not suitable for children under 5 years of age.

trans fat
The ideal intake of trans fat is zero.

micronutrients
Vitamins and minerals are essential for health but only very small amounts are required by the body so they are known as 'micronutrients'.

Vitamins

Vitamins are nutrients that are essential for bodily health. Only small amounts are needed so they are known as micronutrients. Vitamins can be divided into two groups:

▓ Fat-soluble vitamins A, D, E and K.

▓ Water-soluble vitamins B group and C.

beta-carotene can be converted by the body into vitamin A. The body can regulate the conversion rate so no more is converted than needed.

Good sources of beta-carotene include carrots, sweet potato, red peppers, tomatoes, dark green leafy vegetables e.g. broccoli and spinach, yellow fruits e.g. apricots and mangoes.

Fat-soluble vitamins

Small amounts of these vitamins are needed to maintain good health. They are stored in the liver and fatty tissue when not in use so it is possible to build up a reserve. However, it is important not to eat too many very rich sources regularly over an extended period. For example, toxic levels of vitamin A will build up in the body in the unlikely event that liver is eaten every single day for a few weeks.

Animal livers are the richest source of vitamin A in the diet, containing up to 80 times more vitamin A than other food sources. Don't give liver to a child more than once a week. It is also important when taking a supplement containing vitamin A, such as cod liver oil, not to exceed the manufacturer's recommended dose.

Fat-soluble vitamins	Function	Good sources
Vitamin A	Helps maintain the health of skin, strengthens immunity from infections and is essential for vision especially in dim light.	Liver, oily fish, egg yolk, milk, cheese, butter.
Vitamin D	Regulates the amount of calcium and phosphate in the body needed to keep bones and teeth healthy.	Oily fish, egg yolk, fortified foods such as margarine and some breakfast cereals. Most is produced by the body with the action of sunlight on the skin.
Vitamin E	Helps protect cell membranes and supports the immune system by acting as an antioxidant. Also important for healthy nerves and muscles.	Avocado, almond, walnut, wheat germ, nuts, oatmeal, sunflower oil, some margarines, green leafy vegetables, sweet potato, butternut squash.
Vitamin K	Helps wounds heal properly because it is needed for clotting. Needed to help build strong bones.	Green leafy vegetables such as broccoli, spinach, cabbage and parsley, liver, eggs, fish oils and dairy products. Also made by bacteria in the intestine.

Water-soluble vitamins

These vitamins dissolve easily in water and so are lost with urination. A regular intake is important.

Water-soluble vitamins	Function	Good sources
Vitamin B_1 (Thiamin)	Works with other B group vitamins to help break down and release energy from food. Helps keep nerves and muscle tissue healthy.	Pork, offal (organ meats), peas, fresh and dried fruit, wholegrain breads and cereals, some fortified breakfast cereals.
Vitamin B_2 (Riboflavin)	Helps keep skin, eyes and the nervous system healthy; helps produce red blood cells.	Milk, poultry, meat, fish, asparagus, broccoli, spinach, fortified breakfast cereals.
Vitamin B_3 (Niacin)	Helps produce energy from food; helps keep both the nervous and digestive system healthy.	Meat in general, oatmeal, rice, wheat.
Vitamin B_6 (Pyroxidine)	Allows the body to use and store energy from protein and carbohydrates; helps the formation of haemoglobin (the substance that carries oxygen around the body).	Pork, poultry, liver, kidney, fish and eggs, soya beans, oats, potatoes, wholegrains, wheatgerm, peanuts, fortified cereal products.
Folic acid (also known as folate)	Works together with B12 to form healthy red blood cells. During pregnancy it helps reduce the risk of neural tube defects such as spina bifida in unborn babies.	Liver, eggs, broccoli, brussels sprouts, asparagus, peas, citrus fruits, apricots, chick peas, wheat germ.
Vitamin B_{12} (Cyanocobalamin)	Helps make red blood cells and keeps the nervous system healthy; helps release energy from food; needed to process folic acid.	Most meats; salmon, cod, cheese, eggs, yeast extracts and some fortified breakfast cereals. Also produced in small amounts by harmless bacteria in the gut.
Vitamin C	Keeps the immune system strong by its action as an antioxidant. Needed for wound healing and blood clotting. Helps the body absorb iron from vegetables and cereals (non-meat sources).	Citrus fruits, kiwi fruit, berries, mango, strawberries, blackcurrants, broccoli, spinach, brussels sprouts, tomatoes, peppers, parsley, potatoes.

Minerals

The body requires a whole range of dietary minerals, in very small quantities. The following are some main ones.

Minerals	Function	Good sources
Iron	Helps make red blood cells which carry oxygen around the body. Important during periods of rapid growth. Needed for a strong immune system.	Liver, kidney, beef, lamb or mutton, pork, ham, bacon and products from these meats e.g. beef burger, black pudding, pâté, sausage; tinned sardines, turkey (dark meat); eggs, baked beans, whole grains, dried fruit, fortified breakfast cereal.
Calcium	Essential for healthy bones and teeth. Regulates muscle contraction, including the heartbeat. Makes sure blood clots normally. Needed for the efficient functioning of the immune system.	Milk and dairy products, tinned fish.
Zinc	Helps with the healing of wounds, the processing of carbohydrate, fat and protein, and the making of new cells and enzymes.	Red meat, poultry (especially dark meat), fish, shellfish, whole grain cereals, nuts and seeds.
Selenium	Plays an important role in the immune system's function; acts as an antioxidant preventing damage to cells and tissues.	Fish, shellfish, red meat, poultry, whole grains, eggs, garlic, brazil nuts, sesame seeds.
Magnesium	Helps turn food into energy. Important for bone health. Needed for antibody production.	Green leafy vegetables, root vegetables, egg yolks, whole grains, dried fruit.
Potassium	Controls the balance of fluid in the body, may also help lower blood pressure.	Bananas, oranges, tomatoes, peas, beetroot, mushrooms, potato, milk.

Probiotics

Although probiotics are much discussed in the media, and a great deal of research is being carried out in the area, the jury is still out as to whether and how beneficial to health they are. In essence, probiotics are 'good' bacteria which may help fight infection.

Probiotics are familiar to most people in their yogurt form. Popular brands include: 'Everybody/Everykid' by Yoplait, 'Actimel' and 'Activia' by Danone, 'Yakult', 'Muller Vitality' and 'Glenisk organic yogurt'. They are also available in milks, in tablet form or dried form.

What are 'good' bacteria?

Before birth the gastrointestinal tract (from mouth to anus) is sterile (free from any bacteria). Within hours of birth bacteria quickly colonise or attach themselves to the gut. Most of these bacteria come from the birth canal of the mother. The gastrointestinal tract soon contains about 10 times as many bacteria as there are cells in the body.

Although bacteria are generally associated with infection most of the bacteria in the gut are harmless. The majority play important roles in the body, one of which is to boost immunity. In contrast, bacteria that are disease-causing are called 'pathogens'.

Over time the amounts of 'good' bacteria in the gut can change due to gastrointestinal bugs, consumption of antibiotics and many other causes.

The theory behind probiotics is that taking more of these 'good' bacteria may improve the health of the gut and boost immunity. There are a number of different species or strains of these 'good' bacteria and different products contain different ones. They tend to start with names like 'lactobacillus' and 'bifidobacterium'.

'Good' bacteria improve immunity and protect the gut from more harmful bacteria (pathogens) by:

- Secreting antibacterial substances.
- Competing for space in the gut, preventing pathogens latching on.
- Competing for nutrients needed by pathogens for survival.
- Reversing some of the consequences of infection in the lining of the gut.

Probiotics may also be capable of regulating the immune system and the allergic immune cell response of the body.

probiotics

The World Health Organisation and Food and Agriculture Organisation of the United Nations define probiotics as 'live micro-organisms which, when administered in adequate quantities, confer a health benefit to the host'. This translates as: 'Probiotics are bacteria that are alive which, when given in high enough amounts, are beneficial to health.'

probiotics may protect against illness

Studies carried out on children in day care in Finland and Israel found some evidence that children taking probiotics had less illness than those who did not.

more evidence needed
more evidence needed

'Considerably more supporting evidence beyond what is currently provided in the literature' on the benefits of giving probiotics to children 'is required as numerous fundamental questions remain unanswered'. Journal of Pediatric Gastroenterology and Nutrition (October 2006)

So what is the evidence to support giving probiotics to children?

There is good evidence that giving probiotics may prevent diarrhoea when taking antibiotics and reduce the length of an episode of infectious diarrhoea.

There is some evidence that probiotics may reduce the risk of getting a gastrointestinal bug and of contracting respiratory illness in the community setting (for example, daycare) and that they may treat or prevent atopic dermatitis (eczema). The most researched strain of probiotics is LGG which is found in Yoplait Everybody and Avonmore probiotic milk.

Omega-3

Omega-3 is a type of oil, or more specifically a polyunsaturated fat, which has been found to have a number of health benefits. There has been much discussion of it in the media and there has been lots of focus on foods containing omega-3 and their claimed health benefits. A number of products with added omega-3 are now available in the supermarket including eggs, milk and orange juice. Omega-3 supplements are also available in capsule and liquid form.

Most of the health benefits associated with omega-3 come from the fats EPA (eicosapentaenoic acid) and DHA (docosahexaenoic acid). They are found in oily fish such as salmon, sardines and mackerel.

Another omega-3 fat, ALA (alpha-linolenic acid) can be converted by the body into EPA and DHA. ALA is found in nuts, seeds and their oils. However, it may be difficult for the body to convert ALA so it is best to include foods rich in EPA and DHA in the diet.

products enriched with omega-3

are now widely available (often expensive though). Milk, yogurts, orange juice, spreads, mayonnaise all with added omega-3 and eggs laid by chickens fed on omega-3-enriched grain are available. Foods enriched with fish-based rather than plant-based omega-3 seem to be more effective sources of omega-3.

Rich sources of omega-3 fats

- *ALA* Flaxseed oil, rapeseed oil, walnuts
- *EPA and DHA* Oily fish: tuna (fresh or frozen), herring, trout (rainbow), sardines, mackerel, salmon (fresh or tinned), other seafood: pilchards, shrimp, crab and dogfish.

What are the health benefits associated with omega-3 oils?

Omega-3 oils are important for the development of babies' brain, eye and nervous systems during pregnancy and early infancy. They reduce inflammation and help prevent certain chronic diseases such as heart disease and arthritis. Research is going on into other potential benefits omega-3 oils may hold for our health.

How to provide more omega-3 in the diet

Oily fish—tuna (fresh or frozen), herring, trout (rainbow), sardines, mackerel, salmon (fresh or tinned) and other seafood—pilchards, shrimp, crab and dogfish—are a rich source of omega-3. They also provide protein, vitamin D and iron and are a very healthy food. The typical Irish diet is low in oily fish; ideally the family should eat oily fish each week.

Ways to include oily fish in your child's diet

- Get your child used to eating oily fish when young by including it with favourite foods e.g. with jacket potatoes, pizza or pasta dishes.
- Salmon is a popular fish with children as it is one of the milder tasting oily fish.
- Fish can be lightly steamed and served with vegetables and potatoes or added to stir-fries, made into fish cakes and other fish dishes such as fish pie.
- Try to buy organically farmed salmon or wild salmon if available.
- Fresh tuna can be grilled, made into fish cakes, or combined with vegetables and pasta or rice.
- Mackerel may have too strong a flavour for some children; so it may be best if it is combined with other fish or flavours.
- Ensure all bones are removed from fish before serving, but teach your child to check for bones him or herself.
- Avoid buying fish in batter (batter can be high in fat); if you can't get fresh fish buy it frozen without a coating or topping.
- Keep tinned salmon, mackerel, or sardines in the kitchen press ready for a quick meal (tinned tuna usually has lost most of its omega-3 content). You don't have to worry about the bones in tinned fish, as they are usually soft and provide a great source of calcium.
- Eat fish yourself. Children tend to copy their parents' eating habits—if they see you eating and enjoying fish they are more likely to try it themselves.

Keep fish refrigerated until you need to use it. If stored properly, fresh fish should last a day or two after purchase. All fish can be frozen, but oily fish should be used within 3 months of freezing.

Tip Store fish on ice-cubes in the coldest part of the fridge.

omega-3 and behavioural disorders

There is speculation that since omega-3 fats are very concentrated in the brain they may be important for brain function. A lot of research has been done on omega-3 and children who have autism or autistic-spectrum disorders and children who have ADHD and other behavioural disorders. Results have shown that giving these children extra omega-3 may improve their behaviour, learning and/or concentration. Most famous is the Oxford-Durham study which showed improvements in spelling and reading in children with dyspraxia (difficulties carrying out co-ordinated movements or tasks) after being supplemented with omega-3 fats. To date there is no evidence that omega-3 oil supplements help a healthy child's brain power and concentration.

recommended weekly intake of oily fish

From 7 months of age, aim to include two portions (30 g each) of oily fish in the diet per week. A portion size for a 1–3-year-old is 30 g (cooked fish), and for 3–5-year-olds is 60 g. *Note* A cooked salmon steak is about 100 g.

owing to pollution in the seas, fresh tuna should not be given to your child more than once a week. Tinned tuna should not be eaten more than twice a week. Swordfish, shark and marlin may contain concentrated levels of mercury, so should be avoided by all children.

Guidelines for supplements

There are no specific recommendations on supplements but if you wish to give your child a fish oil supplement rather than oily fish here are some guidelines.

- The target dose for most children (over 1 year old) is around 500 mg EPA daily. Don't give more than 900 mg EPA per day.
- Check the label for EPA and DHA, (EPA is more strongly linked with improvements in behaviour, learning and mood in the research studies to date). Some ordinary fish oils, cod liver oil in particular, do not provide very much EPA or DHA. Be sure to check the label.
- A large range of omega-3 supplements are available, but not all are of good quality. They may not only be ineffective but also contain residues of heavy metals such as mercury or other fat-soluble contaminants.
- Check for vitamin E, it is usually found in the good quality supplements. It may protect the fat from breakdown.
- Supplements vary in strength, so check how much a single capsule contains and the number of capsules required each day to achieve the target dose of 500 mg EPA. You don't want your child to have to swallow 15–20 capsules every day!
- It is better to buy capsules rather than liquid fish oil as the EPA and DHA are highly perishable and are destroyed very easily by light, heat and air. They can be destroyed as soon as the bottle is opened even if manufacturer's instructions for storage are followed. If your child is unable to take capsules, break the capsules open as needed and add the contents to any food or drink. Don't heat the food after adding the supplement.
- Don't exceed the manufacturer's recommended dose.

Note Don't assume that low-cost supplements are good value.

What about vegetarians and vegans?

Vegetarians and vegans can get omega-3 oils in walnut oil, rapeseed oil and linseed oil. There are also supplements available containing DHA from sea-algae in health food stores.

For more information on giving omega-3 oils to vegetarians see Chapter 14.

Reliable sources of information

It is important to take care about the source of nutritional information. From 31st October 2016, all properly qualified dietitians in Ireland must be state registered with the Health and Social Care Professionals Council 'CORU', which means that they have been assessed as being qualified to practice. CORU is Ireland's multi-profession health regulator. On the CORU website – www.coru.ie – you can access the Dietitian's Register to check that a dietitian is state registered. Once you have confirmed that the dietitian you are seeing is state registered you can be happy that the advice and information you have received is reliable.

Unfortunately this is not the case for nutritionists. Anyone can set themselves up as a 'nutritionist' and advise people on diet without any qualifications whatsoever. There are more unqualified 'nutritionists' practicing in Ireland than there are qualified.

While the terms nutritionist and dietitian are often interchanged, generally dietitians are specifically trained to give dietary advice to both healthy and sick people and nutritionists are qualified to advise healthy people only. This is because dietitians study medicine as part of their training.

While giving inaccurate dietary information to adults can have serious consequences, children are even more vulnerable. We have witnessed a number of incidents when parents have been given reckless nutritional advice by unqualified nutritionists resulting in their children becoming very unwell. Be very careful who you allow to advise you on your child's diet. Bear in mind that health food shops are generally not qualified to advise you on nutritional issues relating to children.

Don't assume that because you paid a lot of money for a service the person advising you is qualified. In fact the opposite is generally true. A number of times, our service (which is free in the health service) has been shunned for that of a 'nutritionist' with questionable qualifications who charged the earth. If you are seeing a properly qualified dietitian privately it should cost approximately €70–100 for the first visit and no more (at the time of this book going to print).

The dietitian you are seeing is properly qualified if:

He or she is state registered with CORU. The Dietitians' Register on the CORU website – www.coru.ie – contains the names of all dietitians in Ireland who are state registered. It is illegal for a person to call him- or herself a dietitian unless he or she is state registered.

2 Breastfeeding your baby

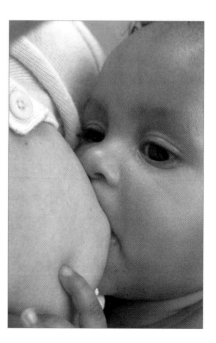

Breast milk is unique. No other milk is so perfectly suited to the nutritional needs of babies. As well as providing the nutrition a baby needs in the first 6 months of life, breast milk contains hundreds of non-nutrient substances that provide protection against common childhood illnesses and enhance the development of the baby's gut, brain and immune system.

While breast milk cannot guarantee perfect health, breastfed babies enjoy better health than their bottle-fed counterparts. It is simply not possible for infant formula in bottle feeds to match the many benefits of breast milk.

Breastfeeding has health benefits for mothers as well as babies and is a very rewarding and satisfying experience for both.

However, while most women can breastfeed, bodies are complicated and sometimes don't work as expected. Good nutrition is vital for your baby's growth and development and if your otherwise well baby is clearly not thriving at the breast, even though you are receiving appropriate help and following good advice, you may have to stop breastfeeding or offer a combination of breast milk and formula milk.

Don't worry if you end up bottle-feeding your baby; be confident in the knowledge that at all times you have your baby's best interests at heart and that bottle-fed babies also thrive and develop well.

The benefits of breastfeeding

Research from Europe, North America and other developed countries has shown that breastfeeding has many health benefits for both babies and mothers.

Breastfed babies

- Have fewer episodes of diarrhoea.
- Have significantly fewer ear infections.
- Have less severe chest infections.
- Are less likely to suffer from certain allergic disorders e.g. eczema, asthma.

There is some, as yet inconclusive, evidence that breastfeeding may protect against sudden infant death syndrome (SIDS) and type 1 diabetes and that breastfed babies may be less likely to become obese. There is also some evidence that babies who are exclusively breastfed for 6 months are less likely to develop leukaemia.

Breastfeeding mothers

- Lose less blood following the birth.
- Wombs return to normal size more quickly.
- Have reduced risk of breast cancer.
- May have reduced risk of ovarian cancer.*

*Results from some research studies have been promising but further studies are needed to prove a definite link.

a rewarding experience

The psychological benefits of breastfeeding are just as important as the benefits to health — it is a very close, emotional and rewarding experience for both mother and baby.

Breastfeeding is also by far the easiest way to feed your baby

- Breast milk is always readily available.
- Breast milk is always at the right temperature—there's no need for bottle warmers.
- There's no need to bring bottles of formula or worry about germs on trips away from home.
- There's no need to sterilise or make up bottles.
- Last, but not least, breast milk is free!

Breastfeeding even for a short period is extremely beneficial to children. Breastfeeding for as little as 13 weeks bestows health advantages that continue throughout childhood into adolescence and beyond.

baby friendly hospitals

The Baby Friendly Hospital Initiative (BFHI) was set up by the World Health Organisation and the United Nations Children's Fund (UNICEF) in 1989. This global initiative promotes, protects and supports breastfeeding.

Hospitals are awarded baby-friendly status if they can show that they are committed to promoting and supporting breastfeeding. To achieve the award hospitals need to have very high and internationally recognised standards. Nearly every maternity hospital in Ireland either has or is seeking to obtain this award.

It is a good idea to check whether your maternity hospital has received baby-friendly status. However, sometimes new or inexperienced staff may be unfamiliar with best practices and if you are unhappy with any aspect of care or are in need of further help and support, it may help to speak with a more senior member of staff. A hospital only deserves its BFHI award if you leave feeling happy and confident about breastfeeding.

Nutrients in breast milk

Breast milk provides nearly all the nutrients your baby needs in the first 6 months of life including protein, carbohydrate, minerals and vitamins, with the exception of vitamins D and K which need to be provided separately.

Once the baby is born, and the placenta (afterbirth) has been delivered, levels of the hormone prolactin start to rise in the mother's blood stream. Prolactin stimulates milk production, by working on the breasts 'telling them' to make milk.

Colostrum

For the first few days the breasts produce colostrum, a yellow-coloured fluid. It is yellow because of its high levels of beta-carotene which converts to vitamin A, an important anti-oxidant which boosts the immune system. Breast milk proper is produced when the milk 'comes in' a few days after the birth.

Colostrum is a very valuable fluid, extremely rich in proteins and antibodies. Some mothers who decide not to breastfeed give their babies colostrum and this confers considerable health benefits on their babies. The amount of colostrum produced is variable.

jaundice

is very common in newborn babies, particularly sleepy babies who are reluctant to feed. It can affect up to 50 per cent of babies and is more common in breastfed babies. It usually develops within 3–5 days of birth and clears once feeding has been established. It may take a little longer to clear in premature babies.

Some babies need phototherapy, in which a special type of light is emitted which helps the baby's body to break down bilirubin, the cause of jaundice. A jaundiced baby needs to breastfeed frequently. Sometimes it is necessary to express the colostrum/breast milk and offer it to the baby from a cup. Your midwife will let you know if this is needed and will show you how to do it.

to achieve baby friendly status maternity hospitals must

- Help mothers initiate breastfeeding soon after birth. Ideally mothers should be helped to initiate breastfeeding within half an hour of the birth. Skin to skin contact is recommended and the baby should be held for at least 30 minutes. Skin to skin contact helps to keep the baby warm and calm, helps regulate the baby's breathing and heart rate and helps with the first breastfeed.
- Show mothers how to breastfeed—breastfeeding is a skill that needs to be acquired by both mother and baby.
- Give newborn babies no food or drink other than breast milk, unless medically indicated.
- Practice rooming in—mothers and infants should be allowed to remain together for 24 hours a day.
- Encourage breastfeeding on demand.
- Give no artificial teats or dummies to breastfeeding infants.

Note In the case of unwell babies medical care takes precedence over any of the above recommendations.

the composition of breast milk
During the 14 days following the birth, the composition of breast milk changes from colostrum (1–5 days) to transitional breast milk and by day 14 or so to mature breast milk. The composition of breast milk is continuously changing to meet the needs of the growing baby.

Colostrum has three very positive effects on the newborn baby's gut:

1 Its antibodies stick to the baby's gut like a protective coating and prevent harmful bacteria from attaching.
2 It contains a special growth factor which stimulates the development of the gut. Babies' guts are a little 'leaky' at birth and colostrum promotes gut closure. It is important that the baby take the first feed within a few hours after birth as this period is a critical window of opportunity for promoting gut closure.
3 It has a mild laxative effect which helps the baby to pass meconium (new-born stools).

Protein

The baby's requirement for protein is highest in the first months of life. The protein concentration in breast milk reduces over subsequent months, balancing perfectly the amount of protein that the baby needs against the amount received from breast milk.

Mature breast milk is lower in protein than infant formula so breastfed babies receive slightly less protein than bottle-fed babies and this is thought to be the reason why breastfed babies have a slightly slower rate of weight gain. There is evidence from medical research that this lower protein intake and slower rate of weight gain may have important long-term health benefits including lower blood pressure and a reduced risk of heart disease and obesity in later life.

Breast milk protein is mostly whey protein and exactly meets the needs of the baby. Whey protein produces a soft curd in the stomach and is more easily digested than casein protein. The whey protein in breast milk also contains a number of anti-infective agents.

Although whey-dominant formula for bottle-feeding is available the whey protein it contains is different to the type found in breast milk and does not contain any anti-infective agents. Casein-dominant and soya-based infant formulas are even less like breast milk.

if your baby is not thriving
A baby who is not thriving may have an underlying medical condition and should always be seen by a doctor.

Fat

Fat is the main energy source for newborn infants. It accounts for 40–50 per cent of total calories in human milk. This high fat content is vital in supporting the baby's rapid growth; it also plays a crucial role in brain development.

There are numerous differences between the fat found in human milk and that in infant formula. Breast milk also contains digestive enzymes which enhance the ability of the baby's gut to digest fat.

Carbohydrate

The main carbohydrate in breast milk is *lactose*, the naturally occurring sugar in milk. It supplies over 35 per cent of the baby's energy needs. Lactose is a combination of two sugars: *glucose* and *galactose*. During digestion lactose is readily broken down into these two sugars. Glucose is essential for the developing brain and galactose is important for the developing nervous system.

Lactose also aids the absorption of calcium and iron and encourages the growth of good bacteria, such as lactobacillus, in the baby's gut.

Minerals

The minerals in breast milk are more easily absorbed than the minerals in formula. Minerals are less influenced by the breastfeeding mother's diet than vitamins.

bioavailability is a measure of how easily the body can absorb nutrients. The bioavailability of minerals in breast milk is high.

Vitamins

Breast milk contains a complete range of vitamins with the exception of vitamins K and D (see below). Water-soluble vitamins, which include all the B vitamins and vitamin C, are well provided in breast milk but their levels can be influenced by the mother's diet so it is important to eat a healthy balanced diet. Babies of vegan breastfeeding mothers are particularly at risk of vitamin B_{12} deficiency (see Chapter 14, page 203).

Vitamin K plays an essential role in blood clotting. It is normally made by bacteria present in the gut. However, it can be some time before these bacteria are fully established in the gut of a new-born infant. All babies (both breast- and formula-fed) are now given a vitamin K injection at birth to build up their stores and to eliminate the risk of haemorrhagic disease, a serious threat to newborns.

Vitamin D

Vitamin D is very important for bone health as it plays a key role in calcium metabolism and bone formation. New scientific findings show that vitamin D has several other very important roles in the body. Deficiency of Vitamin D has been linked with diseases such as asthma, diabetes, multiple sclerosis, certain types of cancer and even dental caries.

It is important for a mother to have good vitamin D stores during pregnancy as this will ensure the baby receives goods levels of vitamin D to build up his or her own store before birth. This store of vitamin D is important because mature breast milk has very low levels of this vitamin. Worryingly, studies have shown that many adults, teenagers and pregnant women living in Ireland have poor vitamin D stores.

National programmes promoting vitamin D supplementation for babies have been in place for several years in the UK, Canada, USA, Australia, Norway, Sweden and the Netherlands. In 2007 the Food Safety Authority of Ireland made a recommendation that Ireland also should have a national policy on supplementing babies with Vitamin D and that all babies, both breastfed and bottle fed, from birth to 12 months, should receive a vitamin D supplement of 5 micrograms per day. This recommendation was endorsed by the Department of Health and Children in 2010.

Suitable vitamin D supplements for infants currently available on the Irish market include Abidec Vitamin D3 Drops, Baby Vit D3 and Baby D. These products are not available on the medical card or the drug payment scheme. They are available to purchase in pharmacies, some supermarkets and other outlets. It is very important to read the information on the label as the number of drops required to provide the recommended 5 micrograms of vitamin D differs for each product. Very high amounts (5 times the recommended dose) of vitamin D are harmful.

A multivitamin containing Vitamin D is not recommended. If your doctor has already prescribed vitamins for your baby you should ask their advice before giving your baby any additional vitamin products.

exclusive breastfeeding

means giving the baby breast milk alone (including expressed breast milk given in a bottle) — no other drinks or food are given. The World Health Organisation recommends exclusive breastfeeding for 6 months, followed by breastfeeding in combination with suitably nutritious solid foods until 2 years of age or older. This has been proven to reduce the risk of respiratory infections, including pneumonia, and ear infections.

Diagnosing Vitamin D deficiency

It is not easy to spot the signs of mild vitamin D deficiency. A more severe case can lead to the development of rickets. Young children with rickets can have deformed bones. A very common feature of this disease is bow legs. The simplest and most effective way of checking for a mild vitamin D deficiency is to have a blood test. If you are worried that you may have poor vitamin D levels you should speak to your GP about getting your levels checked. If you or your baby are found to have very low vitamin D levels a higher dose of vitamin D may be needed.

iron

Babies are born with good stores of iron which last for 5–6 months. Once these stores run out, milk alone will no longer meet the baby's requirement for iron so all babies need to start solids at 6 months of age. It is important that the weaning diet includes iron-rich foods. Iron-deficiency anaemia is probably the most common nutritional disease in toddlers.

Factors affecting the body's vitamin D levels

Sun exposure For most people, sun exposure is the main way of getting vitamin D, which is made by the action of sunlight on the skin. However, the further we live from the equator, the less sunlight we receive and the less vitamin D the skin makes. In Ireland we make little or no vitamin D during the 6 months of the year from October to March. Women who cover up for religious reasons, for example, some Moslem women, receive very little sunlight and are at high risk of vitamin D deficiency.

With growing awareness of the dangers of sun exposure and skin cancer, more and more people are choosing to wear sun screen protection during time spent outdoors. Indeed, many makeup products and moisturisers now contain in-built sun screens which prevent the skin from making vitamin D.

To synthesise vitamin D during the summer months people with fair skin need 15 minutes a day of sunlight exposure to the face and hands. Babies' skin should not be exposed to the sun.

Skin colour It takes dark skin longer to make vitamin D than fair skin (10–50 times longer). This, combined with the weaker sunlight in countries such as Ireland, Britain and Canada which are far north of the equator, increases the risk of vitamin D deficiency in women who are dark skinned.

Diet Foods containing vitamin D include oily fish, eggs, fortified margarines, fortified milks such as Avonmore Supermilk, Goldenvale Supermilk and Dawn Hi & Lo, and some fortified breakfast cereals.

Bioactive compounds in breast milk

Newborn babies have immature immune systems. Breast milk contains a number of bioactive compounds which work to protect them in the first months of life while their own defences are developing.

Anti-microbial factors

Good bacteria in the baby's gut makes it more difficult for harmful bacteria to attach to the gut wall. Breast milk contains factors, e.g. bifidus factor, which promote the growth of good bacteria, including bifidobacteria, in the baby's gut.

Breast milk contains lactoferrin which kills certain bacteria. It also binds to iron which makes it unavailable for harmful bacteria such as E-coli. E-coli cannot grow without readily available iron.

Antibodies protect the baby against harmful bacteria that cause respiratory and gastro-intestinal infections. Breastfed babies receive their mother's own antibodies through breast milk. Levels of antibodies are highest in colostrum but breast milk continues to contain substantial concentrations of antibodies throughout the first 2 years.

Special fat globules, antivirals, present in breast milk have been shown to protect against rotavirus, the leading cause of gastroenteritis in children under 2 years of age.

The levels of lysozyme, a bacteria-killing enzyme, in breast milk are 3000 times those in cow's milk. The levels rise steadily to reach their peak when the baby is 6 months old.

Anti-inflammatory agents

Inflammation is one of the ways the body reacts to infection. Redness, swelling and pain are all caused by the body's inflammatory response. Anti-inflammatory agents in breast milk include anti-oxidants, such as vitamin C and vitamin A, and enzymes that break down inflammation-causing substances released by the body during an infection.

Growth and development substances

Development-promoting substances in breast milk include nucleotides. These are protein-like substances which have been shown to enhance the baby's developing immune system and to contribute to superior iron absorption. They may also act as growth factors. (See Chapter 4, pages 46–7, for more on nucleotides.)

Fore milk and hind milk

The composition of mature breast milk changes from the start of the feed to the end. At the beginning of a feed breast milk has a high lactose content (lactose is the naturally occurring sugar in milk) and fluid/water content but not very much fat. During the feed the fat content

---

Ireland's breastfeeding rate

Ireland has one of the lowest breastfeeding rates in Europe. Figures from 2013 show that 55.8% of mothers were breastfeeding on discharge from hospital. Across Europe on average nine out of ten babies are breastfed, including almost all babies born in Norway, Sweden and Denmark. By three months, four in ten babies in Ireland are breastfed.

As more and more women become aware of the enormous benefits of breast milk, hopefully breastfeeding will become the social norm in Ireland and breastfeeding mothers will receive all the help and support they need to breastfeed their babies for as long as they wish.

of the milk increases to reach 4–5 times the level present at the beginning. This high-fat milk has more calories and is very satisfying for the baby.

The baby usually starts feeding with a short burst of vigorous sucking and then slows the sucking rhythm to a more even pace. Pauses are uncommon early in the feed but become more frequent as the feed progresses, reflecting the increasing fat content.

The milk produced at the beginning of a feed is called 'fore milk'. Milk produced later in the feed is called 'hind milk'. It is very important that a baby receives both fore milk and hind milk and for this reason should always be allowed to feed on the first breast offered until proper sucking stops. If the baby is still hungry after finishing on the first breast the second breast should be offered.

Breastfed babies feed until their appetite is satisfied. The high fat content in hind milk allows them to recognise when they have taken enough to meet their needs and feel full.

> **introducing solids**
> If your baby seems to be too hungry on breast feeds alone at any stage between 4 months (17 weeks) and 6 months of age you may need to introduce solids but check first with your public health nurse or family doctor.

Diet while breastfeeding

The quality of breast milk is usually good even if the mother is unwell, smokes or is eating a less than ideal diet. This is because the body generally favours the breast milk over the wellbeing of the breastfeeding mother. However, vegetarian and vegan breastfeeding mothers need to pay special attention to their diets and may need to take supplements (see Chapter 14).

Do I need to eat extra calories?

There is no need to eat very much more than usual. Only 350–450 extra calories are needed per day. Around 2.7–3.6 kg (6–8 lbs) of body fat is laid down during pregnancy to supply energy for breast milk production after the baby is born. Breastfeeding mothers have also been shown to have a more efficient metabolism meaning that their bodies are better able to conserve energy and 'subsidise' the cost of their milk production. The best advice is to eat to appetite.

How important is a healthy balanced diet?

If your own diet is not ideal the quality of your milk will usually be maintained but at the expense of your own health and wellbeing. Vegetarian and vegan breastfeeding mothers usually need to take supplements. It is important to try and eat well.

- Aim to eat at least 5 portions of fruit and vegetables (fresh, frozen, dried, tinned or a glass of juice) every day.

- Include fibre-rich foods in your diet such as brown bread, pulses, high-fibre breakfast cereals, fruit and vegetables.
- Eat starchy foods such as bread, pasta, rice and potatoes, to give you energy.
- Eat protein-rich foods, such as lean meat and chicken, fish, eggs and pulses.
- Try to have one hot meal a day.
- Avoid skipping meals.
- Eat 1–2 portions of sea fish every week, including oily fish.
- Keep meals simple so they don't take too long to prepare.

If you are concerned that your diet is poor ask your doctor or pharmacist for advice about taking a vitamin supplement.

Do I need extra calcium?

A breastfeeding mother needs to take 1200 mg calcium a day rather than the 800 mg needed normally. Dairy foods, such as milk, cheese and yogurt, are rich in calcium. If you are unable to achieve 1200 mg calcium a day from your diet alone, check with your pharmacist about taking a calcium supplement.

Aim for 5 servings of calcium-rich foods a day.

One serving of calcium is:
- 1 glass (200 mls) of milk
- 1 pot (125 g) of yogurt
- 1 oz hard cheese

fathers' support

Most fathers, once they are aware of the many benefits to health of breastfeeding for both mother and baby are very supportive of their partner's decision to breastfeed. Other family members should also fully support the decision to breastfeed. It is neither acceptable nor helpful, however well intentioned, to put pressure on a breastfeeding mother to start giving the baby a bottle of formula.

Does breastfeeding promote weight loss?

Exclusive breastfeeding combined with diet and exercise results in more effective weight loss than diet and exercise alone. A moderate weight loss of 1–2 lbs (0.5–1.0 kg) a week is perfectly safe while breastfeeding. Strenuous exercise from 6–8 weeks after the birth will not affect milk production.

Do I need to drink extra fluids?

Your fluid intake will not affect the volume of breast milk produced but it is important to stay well hydrated. An adult needs to take at least 6–8 cups of fluid a day and it is reasonable for a breastfeeding mother to aim for a similar intake. Let your thirst be your guide. However, if you have dark or strong-smelling urine this is a sign that you need to drink more. Some women find it helpful to have a drink every time they breastfeed. The best drinks are water and milk but juice, tea, squash and fizzy drinks are acceptable.

What about caffeine?

Caffeine passes readily into breast milk so you should avoid consuming too much while breastfeeding as it can make your baby a bit jittery. Caffeine is found in coffee, tea, cola and energy drinks, and also in chocolate. Caffeine is also found in certain cold and flu remedies so always check with your pharmacist before taking these.

It is best to limit your intake to no more than 300 mg (5 mugs of tea or 2 mugs of coffee) a day. If you drink filtered or percolated coffee don't make it too strong. You can drink as much as you like of the decaffeinated varieties. If you regularly drink tea or coffee it is probably best to avoid cola and energy drinks altogether.

Drink/food	Caffeine content*
1 mug (250 mls) tea	55 mg
1 mug (250 mls) instant coffee	100 mg
1 mug (250 mls) decaffeinated coffee	less than 5 mg
1 mug (250 mls) filtered or percolated coffee	140 mg
330 ml can cola	40 mg
50 g chocolate bar	5–36 mg (the higher the % of cocoa solids the higher the caffeine content)

* The exact amount will vary according to brewing methods and brands of coffee or tea.

Do I need to avoid certain foods?

The only foods you need to cut down on or avoid altogether now, unlike while pregnant, are certain types of fish.

Oily fish The fat contained in oily fish is very beneficial to health (it is not present in tinned tuna). However, oily fish contains pollutants, some of which pass from the fish into breast milk, so you should limit the amount of oily fish you eat.

- Aim to include 1–2 portions a week—but no more—of oily fish— mackerel, sardines, salmon, trout and/or fresh tuna.
- Don't eat more than 1 fresh tuna steak a week or two 8 oz tins of tuna a week.
- Avoid shark, swordfish and marlin.
- Choose from a wide variety of fish.

flavours in breast milk
Breast milk contains a variety of flavouring substances derived from the mother's diet. The infant recognises flavours and responds to them. Thus, unlike the bottle-fed baby, the breastfed baby is exposed to a variety of tastes from the earliest age. This may lead to a greater acceptance and enjoyment of novel foods later on.

Peanuts and tree nuts In the past the British Medical Council recommended avoiding peanuts and peanut-containing products if your baby was at high risk of developing a food allergy. This recommendation is no longer given as new research has shown that avoidance may actually do more harm than good—see Chapter 13.

Other food allergies It is possible for a breastfed baby to develop a food allergy through allergens such as cow's milk and soya being transmitted in the breast milk but this is extremely rare. See Chapter 13 for more information on allergies.

Does what I eat affect the taste of my milk?

Highly spiced or strong tasting foods affect the taste of breast milk and can unsettle some babies. The best approach is trial and error, observing your baby for any signs of discomfort after you have eaten something strongly flavoured or highly-spiced such as a curry. All babies are different and foods that may unsettle one baby are tolerated perfectly well by another.

alcohol and breastfeeding

It is safer to avoid alcohol completely during the first 6 weeks after your baby is born. Newborn babies are very vulnerable to the effects of alcohol and drinking during this time may also hinder your chances of successful breastfeeding.

Once your baby is a little older it should be safe for you have an occasional drink but always wait for the recommended interval for the alcohol to clear completely from your milk before giving a breast feed. This will ensure that your baby is not exposed to any alcohol.

Remember, too, that just as a single drink may impair a person's ability to drive, excessive alcohol consumption may affect a parent's ability to look after their baby properly.

Drinking alcohol while breastfeeding

Any alcohol you drink passes easily into breast milk at concentrations similar to those found in the blood stream. Alcohol that enters the body must be detoxified by the liver. Infants detoxify alcohol at half the rate of adults and consequently even small amounts of alcohol can be harmful to them.

The levels of alcohol in breast milk, even after moderate consumption, may affect a baby by disrupting sleep patterns, reducing milk intake or causing a dangerous drop in blood sugar levels (hypoglycaemia). Experts disagree as to whether breastfeeding mothers should avoid alcohol completely or may safely consume an occasional drink.

Alcohol is not trapped in breast milk but is constantly removed from the milk by passing back into the blood stream. So if you allow enough time to pass between taking an alcoholic drink and breastfeeding you can be certain that all alcohol has been cleared from your milk and your baby will not be exposed to any alcohol.

It takes between 2 and 2½ hours for 1 drink (e.g. a glass of wine or beer) to clear from a breastfeeding mother's milk, depending on her height and weight. Clearing 2 drinks takes between 4 and 5½ hours, 3 drinks take between 6 and 8 hours. For example, if you weigh 11 stone (70 kg) you will need to allow 2¼ hours for every alcoholic drink you take before breastfeeding your baby.

If you take more than one drink and need to wait several hours before feeding the baby, you may have to express some milk to avoid becoming uncomfortable. All of this milk must be thrown away. Expressing your milk has no effect on the time it takes for the alcohol to clear. (See Chapter 3, pages 33–5 for how to express milk.)

Establishing breastfeeding

3

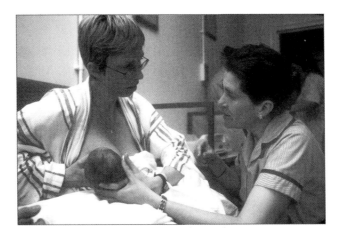

While breastfeeding is perfectly natural, it is still a skill that both mother and baby need to learn. The process of obtaining milk from the breast requires considerably more effort on the part of the baby than drinking from a bottle.

Some babies and mothers will take to breastfeeding very easily whereas others will need a little more time, help and guidance. Good advice from your midwife, lactation consultant (see pages 32 and 41), public health nurse or an experienced friend can make all the difference.

(see pages 32 and 41)

support services

It is a good idea to identify your local health centre before giving birth to find out about the support services available in your area. If possible, get the name of your public health nurse and contact her before the delivery or just after you return home from the hospital. She will visit you at home soon after the birth and on request. It is also possible to see a public health nurse at the weekly baby clinic in your local health centre.

average intake of fluid per feed in the first few days of life

1st day	7 ml
2nd day	14 ml
3rd day	38 ml
4th day	58 ml
5th day	70 ml

The early weeks

Breastfeeding requires time, dedication and commitment. It is quite common for mothers and babies to need a lot of practice before getting breastfeeding right. Don't be afraid to ask for help or guidance from your midwife, public health nurse or lactation consultant. The first couple of weeks may be uncomfortable and very tiring and during this time good family support is vital. Shorter hospital stays mean that many women now find themselves back at home within two days of giving birth.

In the early days while milk supply is being established the baby may need to feed every 2 hours throughout the day and night, allowing very little time for sleep, let alone anything else! It's a big help if somebody else takes care of the shopping, cooking, cleaning, other children etc.

If you intend to breastfeed try to take it as easy as possible for the first 9 or 10 days after the baby is born. This will give you time to recover from the birth and concentrate on feeding your new baby.

Some babies are slow to feed for the first day or two, occasionally for longer. This may be because they are tired, sore or too sedated following the birth. Healthy babies are born with several days' supply of fluid and stored fat (for food) to keep them going until they recover and get hungry.

It is normal for some babies to feed only 3 times (i.e. every 8 hours) during the first 24 hours of life. Babies drink only tiny volumes during the first few days of life, from about 7 ml in the first 24 hours to 70 ml by day 5.

Getting attached

Before starting a breastfeed make sure that you are in a comfortable position and feel relaxed. You can breastfeed while sitting in bed or on a chair, including a suitable armchair, or on a sofa, with your back well supported with cushions.

The first and most important step is to ensure that the baby attaches to the breast properly. The nipple and most of the areola (the brownish or pink ring of tissue surrounding the nipple) should be inside the baby's mouth. Without proper attachment the baby will not be able to get enough milk. Poor attachment is also the most common cause of sore nipples.

It is more difficult for the baby to get colostrum from the breast than breast milk so correct attachment is necessary from the very beginning.

Tips to make sure your baby is attached to the breast correctly

First, position the baby correctly

- Place your baby close to you with his or her head and shoulders turned towards the breast.
- The baby's neck should not be twisted.
- Bring the baby to the breast, rather than the breast to the baby!
- Support the baby's head so that it can be extended slightly on the way to the breast— the chin and lower jaw should reach the breast first.
- The baby's nose and top lip should be directly opposite the nipple.

correct attachment

If the baby is attached correctly there should be no friction of the tongue or gum on the nipple and no movement of the breast tissue in and out of the baby's mouth. The baby's sucking should not damage the nipple and there should be no soreness.

Now brush the baby's mouth against the nipple to trigger the rooting reflex. A baby 'roots' or searches for the breast. This contact is the only way the young baby knows the breast is there.

Once the baby's mouth is open—it should gape wide to accept the breast—move the baby's entire upper body towards the breast with a swift, positive and well-directed action. The nipple and most of the areola should now be inside the baby's mouth.

The baby's jaw should be located well below the base of the nipple and the tongue should also be under the nipple. The baby's jaw and tongue work on the milk ducts of the breast below the nipple to effect milk release.

The baby is well attached when

- More of the areola is covered with the lower than the upper lip, though it may not always be possible to see this.
- The baby's lips are turned outwards but again it may not always be possible to see the bottom lip.
- The baby's chin is touching your breast.
- The baby's body is slightly rotated upwards so that he or she is looking at you.

At the start of a feed, the baby should suck strongly and continuously with very few pauses. Most mothers are surprised at the strength of the baby's sucking action. As the feed progresses and the fat content of the milk increases, making the milk more satisfying, the baby's sucking will slow down to long deep sucks with more pauses.

Feeding should always be led by the baby who may not want to feed on the second breast or may feed on the second breast for as long as on the first. Your baby will usually let you know what he or she wants. It's usually easy to recognise, especially when a baby is sleepy and contented after a feed, that he or she has had enough milk. Sometimes it's not so easy but in time, as you get to know your baby better, you will become quite expert at figuring out his or her wants and needs.

detaching your baby
When you are taking your baby off the breast first insert your little finger into the corner of the mouth to break the suction.

Discomforts during the first week

It is normal for mothers to experience the following discomforts during the early days of breastfeeding.

- Increased sensitivity of the nipples.
- Sharp pain in the areola (the pink or brown area of skin around the nipple) at the beginning of feeds.
- Engorgement—when the breast becomes over full.
- Stomach pain—breastfeeding helps your womb to contract and you may experience period-like pain during a breastfeed especially if this is not your first child.

Once breastfeeding is established feeding should not be painful except for a possible twinge at the beginning of feeds. During the feed you should experience a painless drawing sensation.

Cracked and sore nipples

Pain after breastfeeding is established should be taken as a warning sign that something isn't right. If you experience pain while feeding or you develop sore nipples it may be a sign that the baby is not attaching to the breast properly.

Prevention is best. The single most important factor in preventing cracked or sore nipples is to ensure from the very beginning that the baby is latching on to the breast properly. If you do develop sore or cracked nipples seek advice on treatment from your doctor, public health nurse or lactation consultant.

engorgement
This is the stage when the breast has become over full. It is the build up of breast milk between feeds and is common in the early days and weeks. It will settle once breastfeeding has become established. Also, in the first 2–4 days after birth there is increased blood supply to the breasts as they prepare for milk production.

Tongue Tie

There is a fold of skin under the tongue that connects the tongue to the bottom of the mouth. If this fold is too short, it may restrict movement of the tongue. If a baby has restricted tongue movement, this can cause breastfeeding difficulties such as problems 'latching on', sore nipples and poor infant weight gain. A diagnosis of tongue tie should be considered if breastfeeding problems persist despite a review of positioning and attachment by an experienced midwife, public health nurse or other skilled healthcare professional.

An information booklet for parents is available to download from the website www.nice.org.uk/guidance/ipg149/informationforpublic. A lot of very useful information is also available from the website of Lactation Consultant Nicola O'Byrne, at www.breastfeedingsupport.ie.

Thrush

Thrush is a fungal infection which can thrive in warm moist conditions and on broken skin such as cracked nipples. It is characterised by nipple pain which intensifies during a feed and continues for some time between feeds.

good personal hygiene is all that is necessary while breastfeeding. If you use breast pads you should change them frequently, even during the night, as a moist milky environment is the perfect breeding ground for bacteria and fungi. It is not a good idea to use breast pads if you have thrush.

Thrush is more likely to occur following a course of antibiotics. It requires anti-fungal treatment prescribed by a doctor.

If you have thrush you and your baby will both need to be treated at the same time. If your baby has thrush you may notice a white coating on the tongue, gums and inner cheeks, although this is not present in all cases.

Don't store expressed milk during an episode of thrush; it should either be fed to the baby straight away or discarded.

the 'let down' reflex refers to the flow of breast milk in response to the release of the hormone oxytocin when the baby suckles at the breast. The let down reflex varies from woman to woman. In some women it can be quite strong, causing sharp, needle-like pains in the breast and milk may actually spurt from the nipples in jets. Other women experience a tingling sensation and milk may drip from the breast. Some mothers feel nothing at all and milk is only released from the breast by the action of the baby's mouth and tongue. All of these responses are perfectly normal and simply reflect different biological make ups.

As breastfeeding becomes established oxytocin can be released and the milk starts to flow in response not only to the baby suckling at the breast but simply to the sight or sound of the baby — for example, when the baby cries for a feed or even while you are getting ready for a breastfeed.

Mastitis

Mastitis is inflammation of the breast caused by breast milk leaking into the breast tissue. This will only happen if there is a build-up of pressure. The most common cause is the breast not being emptied during feeds because the baby is not correctly positioned at the breast, or is not attaching to the breast correctly or if the baby's feeding is restricted for any reason.

Early signs of mastitis
- Small lump in the breast.
- Appearance of a red patch or red streak on the breast.
- Breast tissue hot and painful to the touch.
- Raised temperature along with aching, flu-like symptoms.

What to do if you have mastitis
- Continue breastfeeding—you may do more harm than good by stopping.
- At the first signs of mastitis feed your baby from the affected breast for as long and as often as the baby is willing.
- Make sure that the baby is correctly positioned and attached as it is very important that the breast is emptied.
- Try different positions during the feed—this may help to empty the breast.
- You may need to express milk in order to empty the breast.
- Place a warm compress on the breast before feeding; this is soothing and may help your milk to flow more easily.
- Very gently massage the breast by stroking the affected area downwards towards the nipple.
- Avoid wearing clothing that puts pressure on the breasts and don't grip the breast tightly when supporting it while feeding.

If the symptoms fail to improve after 12–24 hours of improved milk removal, or if symptoms worsen, it is best to see your GP as the mastitis may have developed into an infection and if so an antibiotic will be needed.

Lactation consultants

Most problems encountered during breastfeeding can be readily resolved with the right advice and support. If you or your baby are having problems breastfeeding while in hospital and you feel that you need more expert advice you should ask to speak to the lactation consultant. These are health care workers (usually nurses) who have attended and passed an internationally certified breastfeeding course. They have invaluable knowledge and experience in dealing with breastfeeding problems.

If you have returned home it may be possible to see the lactation consultant in the hospital outpatients at a drop-in clinic. Many maternity hospitals run these clinics once a week.

While most lactation consultants are hospital based, some work privately and will visit you at home. You should check that the consultant is a member of the Association of Lactation Consultants in Ireland (ALCI). All members of ALCI have been trained to a high standard and have passed the International Board of Certified Lactation Consultants' examination. A home visit costs €60–90 and lasts 1½–2 hours. The fees are refundable on some private health insurance maternity plans. (See page 41 for contact details.)

wind, colic and constipation

Contrary to popular opinion breastfed babies can suffer from all of these problems. (See Chapter 7 for information and advice.)

Feeding your baby expressed milk

In the first days after birth you may need to express some milk if your baby is a slow feeder and you are producing more milk than needed. You can store this expressed milk for use later. Your midwife will teach you how to express milk by hand.

You should probably not give a dummy or bottle while the baby is learning to suckle properly. However, sometime after the first two weeks, once the baby is feeding well from the breast, it can be a good idea to offer a bottle of expressed breast milk once a day, every 3–4 days. This is because it may not always be possible to breastfeed, for example if you become ill or you simply need a break from the unrelenting feeding schedule. The chances are that someone else will be only too glad to feed the baby. Everyone thoroughly enjoys the experience of feeding a small baby.

nipple confusion

It has been suggested over the years that breastfed babies who are offered bottle feeds can become confused between the two different methods of feeding. There is no evidence to support this theory. Admittedly, babies find it easier to drink from a bottle than the breast and if offered bottle feeds too often get lazy and refuse the breast!

If your baby becomes ill with gastroenteritis extra fluids from a bottle may be necessary to maintain hydration.

Feeding from a bottle is completely different to feeding from the breast and some breastfed babies are not keen on accepting milk from a bottle. It can take a number of attempts over several days before they will willingly drink from the bottle. The baby may accept the bottle better from somebody besides the mother. Babies are very sensitive to the sight, smell and sound of their mother as well as the smell of breast milk.

Babies under 3 months old need roughly 100–180 mls (3–6 oz) per bottle feed and babies over 3 months old will take 150–210 mls (5–7 oz) per feed.

When is the best time to express milk?

There is no set ideal time for expressing milk. Every mother is different. It's best to choose the time of day when milk is most plentiful, provided that this time is also convenient for expressing. Most mothers find that their milk supply is at its best in the morning and this tends to be the best time to express. You should express straight after a feed to allow plenty of time for the breasts to fill up again before the next feed is due.

Always wash and dry your hands thoroughly before expressing or handling expressed breast milk.

Breast pumps

It is best to wait until the milk is in and flowing before using electric or hand pumps. It doesn't matter which method of expression you use so long as you find it comfortable, successful and acceptable.

The amount of milk expressed can vary at each expression and from day to day. Electric pumps are usually more effective than manual pumps and might be a better option if you are planning to express on a regular basis. Single and double pumps are available. Double pumping with an electric pump is better if your supply is diminishing or if you need to express more than twice a day for more than a couple of days. It is quicker and encourages an increased milk supply compared with other methods of expression.

Pump models vary in type and quality and what suits one mother may not work as well for another. It is important that whatever pump you choose fits your breast, creating a good but comfortable seal, and produces the right amount of pumping pressure for you.

Different pump models have different vacuum patterns and this pattern is one of the main factors affecting your comfort while expressing. Pumps can be bought in most baby shops or pharmacies.

Storage of expressed breast milk

Expressed breast milk can be kept at room temperature for up to 6 hours. It can be stored in the fridge at a temperature of 2–4 °C for up to 5 days. It is important to store breast milk in the coolest part of the fridge. If the fridge has an inbuilt ice compartment the coolest part is usually the top shelf next to the ice compartment. If it has no ice compartment the coolest part is usually at the back of the bottom shelf. (Check your fridge manufacturer's guidelines.)

If you intend storing your milk for up to 5 days you should buy a refrigerator thermometer. If it is not possible for you to check the temperature of the fridge it is safest to use the milk within 48 hours. Expressed breast milk should not be stored in the door of the fridge.

Breast milk may separate during storage. If this happens just gently shake the bottle to mix the milk again.

Refrigerating breast milk has no effect on its nutrient content. It does, however, reduce some of the protective factors.

Freezing breast milk

You can also freeze the milk. Breast milk can be stored for 2 weeks in the ice compartment of the fridge, or up to 3 months in the freezer section of a fridge freezer with separate doors, or 6 months in a chest freezer. Always store the milk at the back of the freezer. If you have a self defrosting freezer, store the milk as far away as possible from the defrosting element.

When storing milk in a sterile container for freezing don't fill the container to the top. Leave a space of about 2.5 cm or 1 inch from the top as the milk will expand as it freezes.

Freezing breast milk has only minimal effect on the nutrient content but does destroy the protective factors. However, these effects are nothing to worry about as refrigerated or frozen breast milk is still superior to infant formula.

Thawing frozen breast

Frozen breast milk can be thawed slowly in a refrigerator or it can be thawed quickly by placing the container under warm running water. Don't use hot or boiling water as it will destroy anti-infective agents and some vitamins present in the milk. Frozen breast milk should not be thawed at room temperature. To prevent contamination tap water should not be allowed to come into contact with the lid of the container. You will need to swirl the container to mix any layers that have formed.

Breast milk that has been thawed out in the fridge may be stored in the fridge for up to 24 hours before use. Once breast milk has warmed to room temperature it must be used immediately. Breast milk should not be refrozen.

Suitable storage containers

Equipment used in the expressing, handling, storage, and feeding of expressed breast milk must be clean and sterile just as for infant formula. Babies have immature immune systems and you need to take every care not to expose them to bacteria and viruses than can cause illness such as diarrhoea and vomiting. (See Chapter 5, pages 54–7 for more information on cleaning and sterilising equipment.)

Breast milk must always be stored in a sterile air-tight container. Any type of plastic container is suitable provided it has an airtight seal and can be sterilised. Pre-sterilised containers made by Avent are available but the lids are not sterile and must

colour of breast milk

Breast milk is a different colour from infant formula, it may be blue-white (fore milk) or creamy-coloured (higher fat hind milk) and may separate on standing into layers. Breast milk may look 'thin' compared with formula but this is no reflection on its nutritional quality, not to mention all its other properties!

heating expressed breast milk

Before giving a bottle of expressed breast milk to your baby you need to warm it in a jug or bowl of warm water to at least room temperature. Don't use boiling water as this would destroy valuable nutrients. Microwaving breast milk is not recommended as it interferes with the anti-infective properties as well as decreasing the vitamin C content.

feeding expressed milk

Just as with formula for bottle feeds you will need to sterilise the bottles and teats when you feed your baby expressed breast milk.

be sterilised before use. Breast milk storage bags made by Lansinoh or Boots are also convenient. The bags are pre-sterilised and are suitable for immediate use but can be used only once. It is important to date and label each container or bag and always to use the oldest first.

Hand-washing reduces the number of bacteria on the skin but does not get rid of them completely. For this reason great care must be taken not to touch the inside of containers, lids or storage bags.

Support groups

Health centres throughout Ireland run free weekly breastfeeding support groups. They provide an opportunity for pregnant and breastfeeding mothers to meet up for support and advice. Your local health centre will have the details of groups running in your area. Contact your GP or the HSE's Breastfeeding Support Network (1850 241850 www.breastfeeding.ie) for details of your local health centre.

La Lèche League is a voluntary organisation providing information and support to women who want to breastfeed their babies. Volunteer mothers, who have breastfeed their own babies and completed an accreditation programme, provide help and information on breastfeeding at monthly meetings, in person or over the phone. La Lèche League has produced a number of information leaflets which are available free of charge. (See page 41 for contact details)

CUIDIU—Irish Childbirth Trust CUIDIU (the Irish for 'caring support') is a voluntary parent to parent support group. It aims to provide information, education and support on all aspects of parenthood. The group runs a diverse programme of events and activities including breastfeeding support groups. (See page 41 for contact details.)

Breastfeeding while out and about

One of the advantages of breastfeeding is that it gives you great freedom to get out and about and to meet friends and family. If you feel comfortable, confident and at ease it should be possible to breastfeed your baby anywhere—in shops, buses, trains, planes, park benches and restaurants. A baby who is being discreetly breastfed simply appears to be snuggling up against the mother. Some department stores and restaurants provide breastfeeding rooms where you can feed your baby in private if you prefer. In May 2016 a 'Breastfeeding welcome here' mark was launched and is available to all businesses including cafes, restaurants, pharmacies and shopping centres throughout Ireland. Shortly after the launch, several leading businesses agreed to display the mark prominently on their premises and many more are likely to follow.

The Health Service Executive (HSE), in conjunction with the Equality Authority, has a policy of promoting breastfeeding and protecting a mother's right to breastfeed her baby wherever and whenever she wants or needs.

HSE and Equality Authority advice for breastfeeding mothers

- You don't have to ask if you may breastfeed; you can breastfeed anywhere you and your baby want or need to.
- If you are happy to breastfeed in a public area the owner, manager or member of staff of these premises is not allowed to ask you to use separate facilities or ask you to leave.
- Find out if there are any restaurants, shopping centres, hotels or other places in your area that particularly welcome breastfeeding mothers.
- If you would prefer more privacy, ask if the restaurant, hotel or shopping centre has a private feeding room (not a toilet) available for your use.
- If you wear fairly loose-fitting clothing, it will make it easier to be discreet. Most people will hardly even notice that you are breastfeeding.

More information is available from www.breastfeeding.ie or contact the Equality Authority on LoCall 1890 245 545.

Breastfeeding and going back to work

Women in the workforce are entitled to breastfeeding breaks during the working day without loss of pay. This is to facilitate continuation of breastfeeding after the return to work following maternity leave. Maternity leave was increased to 26 weeks in 2007 to help promote exclusive breastfeeding for the first 6 months of life.

Once you return to work your employer is obliged to provide you with a suitable place for expressing milk or feeding your baby during the working day. However, this may not always be possible and if no such space can be provided then you are entitled to a shorter working day, that is the normal working day less the time you are entitled for breastfeeding/expressing.

For information on the arrangements to support breastfeeding in your workplace ask your employer, line manager, human resource staff or union representative. The HSE's guide for parents and employers 'Breastfeeding and Work' can be viewed on www.breastfeeding.ie.

Older babies, of 9 months or more, established on solids, may need only 3 breastfeeds a day. It may be possible to breastfeed your baby before and after work and express just once during the day.

signs of hunger

Intervals between feeds can be unpredictable during the first few weeks. It is better to watch the baby for signs of hunger than to watch the clock. These signs include the baby moving around in a restless way or making sucking motions with the lips and tongue. Hopefully, from around 3 weeks, when milk supply is established, you will be able to get into some sort of feeding routine that works for you and your baby.

non-nutritive sucking

A baby may need to suck on something in order to settle to sleep. It is perfectly fine to offer your baby a dummy if you feel the extra comfort is really needed. You may not need to give it every time the baby is going to sleep. From around 3 months the need to suck in order to settle declines.

fore and hind milk

Fore milk—the milk produced at the beginning of a feed—has a low fat content; this changes during the feed so that the later milk—hind milk—has a high fat content which is very satisfying for the baby. Babies need both fore and hind milk so should be allowed to continue to feed on one breast until it is nearly empty.

your baby's weight gain

During the first 2 weeks after birth it is normal for your baby to lose weight and then return to the birth weight. After this the normal rate of weight gain for a breastfed baby is 150–350 g per week for the first 3 months. Your public health nurse will check your baby's weight when she visits you at home. You can also get your baby's weight checked at the weekly baby clinic in your local health centre.

Frequently asked questions

How long should a breastfeed last?

There is no single answer to this question as mothers and babies vary so much. How long a particular baby needs to breastfeed depends on two factors:

- The rate at which the milk is transferred from the mother to the baby. This rate of transfer varies from mother to mother. In some women the rate can be quite quick whereas in others it is much slower.
- The demand for milk by the baby—a baby who is very hungry may feed quite quickly whereas at other times the feed progresses more slowly.

Some babies may finish feeding in less than 10 minutes but those whose mothers have a slower rate of milk transfer need longer.

It is best to leave the baby to finish on the first breast before offering the second. The sign that the baby is finished is that proper sucking stops. A baby should always be allowed to feed to appetite. It doesn't matter if the baby only feeds from one breast at a single feed—just make sure to start with the other breast at the next feed. You may find it helpful to attach a safety pin or some other marker to your bra strap to remind you which breast to use at the next feed.

Note If a breastfeed regularly lasts longer than 30 minutes per breast you should check that the baby is attaching properly.

How often should my baby breastfeed?

Feeds tend to be infrequent during the first 24–48 hours. A baby may feed as little as 3 times during the first 24 hours. In an otherwise well baby this is perfectly normal.

The feed frequency will increase during the first week of life and often peaks around the fifth day. Some babies may feed every 1½–2 hours (timed from the beginning of one feed to the start of the next) whereas others may leave a longer gap of 3–4 hours between feeds.

During the first weeks of breastfeeding most babies have a period of a few hours when they want to feed every hour. You may find that you are unable to comfort your baby without offering the breast as the baby smells the milk and will root even when well fed. A fussy, breastfed baby who has been well fed may need to be comforted by someone else. Your fatigue and stamina have to be balanced against the needs of your baby.

If feeds are less than an hour apart this may be due to poor intake caused by incorrect attachment at the breast. Or the baby may not be getting enough hind milk (see box on page 38). If you think your baby is not getting enough hind milk it is a good idea to encourage feeding for a little longer on the first breast and see if this helps.

Once established on breastfeeds a baby usually feeds 6–8 times in a 24-hour period. However, if your baby feeds less than 6 times in 24 hours you should wake him or her for feeds.

By the time your baby is 4 months old you may find that 5 breastfeeds a day are sufficient; by 6 months the feeds have usually settled into a pattern of 4–5 times a day. When you drop a feed it will take your body a few days to adapt.

It is best only to feed the baby when he or she is actually hungry, and not always to offer the breast every time the baby cries. Babies cry because they are over-tired, over-stimulated, uncomfortable with wind or colic or have a dirty nappy. Some babies cry when they are trying to go to sleep. Swaddling the baby (see page 95) may also help with settling.

Will my milk supply be enough for the baby?
One of the major reasons that mothers introduce formula or other foods into their baby's diet is that they think they haven't enough milk. They are often mistaken in this as 99 per cent of women are capable of producing enough milk for their babies. Remember that it takes 3–6 weeks to establish breastfeeding.

A mother's ability to produce milk for her baby usually far exceeds anything the baby will need. Be confident that increased demand from your baby will be matched by increased supply from your body. For example, a mother of twins will make twice as much milk as the mother of one baby because there is twice the demand! If you have a contented, growing baby you can be sure that your baby is getting enough milk.

If you are worried that your milk supply is inadequate ask for advice from your midwife, lactation consultant or public health nurse. They should be able to check your breastfeeding technique and advise on a number of practical measures that may help boost milk production.

Is it necessary for me to give feeds at night?
Milk production continues as effectively by night as by day. Indeed, more of the hormone prolactin is released in response to night feeds than day feeds. In the first two weeks of breastfeeding prolactin levels contribute to establishing a good milk supply, so it is important to feed during the night.

signs that your baby may be unwell

A very quiet baby who is sleeping a lot may be weak as a result of not getting enough feed, or may not be interested in feeds because he or she is unwell.

Other signs to watch out for include very few wet nappies (less than 5 in 24 hours) and dark and strong-smelling urine. Small, green-coloured stools can also be cause for concern.

It is best to contact your doctor or public health nurse if you are worried.

milk production

Feeding in itself stimulates milk production: the more you feed the more milk is produced. However, a mother's fatigue can reduce the production of milk. So it is important that you do not become over-tired.

if you can't produce enough milk

A small number of women are not able to produce enough milk despite making every effort to boost milk production. You should not feel bad if this happens: remember that everyone's body is different and sometimes our bodies don't work as well as they should through no fault of our own. The ability of the breasts to produce milk is not influenced by size.

Feeding the baby at night is also necessary to prevent engorgement. It is not a good sign to wake in the morning with an over-full feeling in your breasts. This can result in decreased milk production. Once breastfeeding is established it is all right to miss the occasional night feed but if this is done repeatedly, it is very likely that your milk supply will suffer. Your baby should sleep in the same room as you for at least the first 6 months.

Should I offer extra fluids besides breast milk to my baby?

Breast milk is about 87 per cent water. There is no evidence to suggest that a baby who is breastfeeding well needs extra drinks of water, even in hot climates. If the baby is growing normally then it can almost always be taken for granted that he or she is also receiving enough fluid from breast milk.

factors influencing breast milk production

Once breastfeeding is established there are two main factors that affect the amount of milk produced — frequency of feeding and the mother's fatigue.

The single most important factor determining how much milk is produced is the removal of milk from the breast. In other words, the more you feed the more milk is produced.

Breast milk production closely matches the needs of the baby. As soon as milk is removed from the breasts, milk production automatically restarts in preparation for the next feed. Milk production is at its highest immediately following a feed.

The more milk a baby removes from the breast during a feed, the more milk is made for subsequent feeds.

However, if a baby suddenly demands bigger volume feeds, e.g. during a growth spurt, it can take the breasts a few days to increase production to catch up with the baby's needs. It can be helpful to have a reserve of expressed breast milk always on stand by for times such as these.

If breasts are allowed to become engorged (over full), this reduces milk production and it also makes the release of milk from the breasts more difficult.

The second most important factor influencing milk production is fatigue. Mothers who are extremely tired may find that their milk supply is reduced. Don't hesitate to look for extra help if you need it. Tension or illness may also interfere with milk production.

How do I know when breastfeeding is going well?

- Your baby appears content and satisfied after most feeds.
- Your baby is latching onto the breast properly.
- Your baby is healthy and gaining weight satisfactorily.

- Your baby has at least 6 wet nappies a day.
- Your baby is passing a soft yellow stool as often as after every feed or at least 3 times per day (up to the age of 6 weeks).
- Your breasts and nipples aren't sore.

Useful contacts

Support groups

Association of Lactation Consultants Ireland (ALCI) www.alcireland.ie info@alcireland.ie

CUIDIU Head Office, Carmichael Centre, North Brunswick Street, Dublin 7. Tel (01) 872 4501 for general enquiries; email: info@cuidiu.ie www.cuidiu-ict.ie

Breastfeeding Support Network 1850 241850 www.breastfeeding.ie

For a full list of publications to download or available free of charge see www.healthpromotion.ie

Irish Multiple Births Association gives support and information to parents of 'multiples'. Tel 01 8749056 info@imba.ie www.imba.ie

La Lèche League There are branches throughout Ireland—check your local telephone directory for a La Lèche league leader in your area or log on to La Lèche League's website, www.lalecheleagueireland.com, for full details and contact telephone numbers.

Lactation consultants working in private practice

Cork City Geraldine Cahill Tel 087 8187240 email: gerbaldwincahill@gmail.com

South Dublin and North Wicklow Nicola O'Byrne Tel 086 231 2679 email: info@breastfeedingsupport.ie www.breastfeedingsupport.ie

Other www.alcireland.ie – click on Find a Lactation Consultant

Websites

Baby Friendly Hospital Initiative (BFHI) www.ihph.ie/babyfriendlyinitiative www.babyfriendly.org.uk Locall 1890 245 545

The Equality Authority Tel (01) 417 3333 info@equality.ie www.equality.ie www.rollercoaster.ie. This is a parenting website which includes a discussion forum.

Publication

What to expect when you are breastfeeding and what to do if you can't Clare Byam-Cook, Vermilion, London, revised and updated 2006.

4 Choosing a formula when bottle-feeding your baby

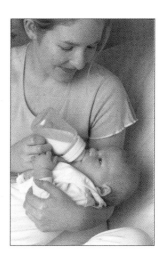

Babies' extraordinarily rapid rate of growth in their first year of life means that they have very high nutritional requirements. For instance, they need more calcium and protein than toddlers and young children. Breast milk best meets the baby's needs but infant formula is an acceptable substitute. No other milk is suitable for babies.

The composition of infant formula has improved dramatically over the past 30 years as research has greatly increased our understanding of breast milk composition and therefore how to manufacture a formula substitute. These efforts continue with the aim of matching infant formula as closely as possible to breast milk. However it will never be possible for infant formula to fully match the unique properties of breast milk.

A wide range of infant formulas is available which can make the choice between them rather confusing. In this chapter we give you information on the composition of various formulas and guidelines on which formula to choose and why. In the following chapter we advise on cleaning and sterilising feeding equipment, on making up and storing feeds and on feeding schedules. We hope that the time spent feeding your baby during this amazing first year of a life is a relaxing and truly enjoyable experience.

First milks and milks for hungrier babies

With rare exceptions (see page 48) cow's milk-based infant formula should be the first choice for feeding healthy babies who are not exclusively breastfed. These formulas are made from extensively modified cow's milk under strictly enforced guidelines.

First milks and milks for hungrier babies, which are based on cow's milk protein, are both suitable for babies from birth up to 12 months old. The main difference between them is the mix of cow's milk protein they contain: first milks are whey dominant and milks for hungrier babies are casein dominant. Whey protein forms a soft curd in the stomach with a consistency like yogurt; casein protein forms a firmer curd in the stomach with a consistency like cottage cheese.

high quality of baby formula

Whether you choose to bottle-feed your baby from the beginning or to supplement breastfeeding with formula it is very reassuring to know that the quality of infant formula is strictly regulated and has improved dramatically over the last 30 years.

Brands of first milks and milks for hungrier babies available on the Irish market

First milks; labelled 'from birth' (whey dominant)	Milks 'for hungrier babies' (casein dominant)
Aptamil First or Profutura First Milk	Aptamil Hungry Milk
Cow & Gate First Infant Milk	Cow & Gate Infant Milk for Hungrier Babies
SMA PRO First Infant Milk	SMA Extra Hungry Infant Milk

The protein in first or whey-dominant milks is 60–70 per cent whey and 30–40 per cent casein. The protein in second milks is 80 per cent casein and 20 per cent whey. The protein combination in first milks more closely matches the protein in breast milk so first milks should be given unless otherwise indicated (see below).

Casein-dominant milk is marketed for the hungrier baby. It has a similar calorie content to whey-dominant (first) milks but casein is more slowly digested than whey and takes longer to leave the stomach, so it is thought that the baby may feel fuller for longer. However, this has not been scientifically proven. If your baby seems excessively hungry it is worth trying a casein-dominant formula.

See Chapter 5, page 62 for a guide to normal feeding patterns and practical advice.

Composition of first milks available on the Irish market

	Cow & Gate First Infant Milk	SMA PRO First Infant Milk	Aptamil First Milk	Aptamil Profutura First Milk
Energy (kcals per 100 mls)	66	67	66	66
Protein (g per 100 mls)	1.3	1.3	1.3	1.3
LCPs (AA & DHA)	Added	Added	Added	Added
Prebiotics	Added	Added*	Added	Added

* Prebiotics are added to the powder formula only and are not present in the ready to feed (liquid) formula

Milk with partially digested protein

Cow & Gate Comfort, SMA Comfort and Aptamil Comfort, marketed as for 'comfortable digestion' are suitable for babies from birth. They contain partially digested (hydrolysed) cow's milk protein, making them different from the other infant formulas. They also have a lower lactose (milk sugar) content and a special type of fat blend. They are not suitable for babies with cow's milk allergy. Although first milks are the best choice for healthy newborn babies Cow & Gate Comfort, SMA Comfort and Aptamil Comfort are marketed for babies with colic, reflux and/or constipation.

If your baby has a persistent problem with constipation, consider a week's trial on Cow & Gate Comfort, SMA Comfort or Aptamil Comfort provided your GP or public health/practice nurse/dietitian agrees. If the constipation improves you should continue giving your baby Cow & Gate Comfort, SMA Comfort or Aptamil Comfort until he or she is taking a wide variety of spoon feeds—usually 2–3 months after beginning weaning when the baby is 6–9 months old.

Follow-on milks

Like milks for hungrier babies, follow-on formulas are casein dominant. However, they have higher levels of iron, protein, calcium and phosphorus than first milks or milks for hungrier babies. Because of this they are not suitable for babies less than 6 months old. This is clearly stated on tins of follow-on formulae at the request of UK and Irish health care professionals.

You should only give follow-on milk if you think your baby's diet may be deficient in iron. A full-term baby is born with a good iron store but this is gradually used up over the first 6 months of life. For this reason it is important that iron-rich foods are included in the weaning diet (see Chapter 6, page 73). If they are not and/or the baby is taking less than 400 mls a day of standard infant formula, a follow-on milk should be given.

unmodified fresh cow's milk

is completely unsuitable for babies under 1 year of age. The protein, calcium and sodium (salt) content in cow's milk is up to 3 times higher than the amounts found in breast milk. A baby's immature kidneys can't cope with such high levels of these nutrients. Unmodified cow's milk is also a very poor source of iron.

protein source

EU Guidelines allow the use of the following protein sources in infant formula

- Cow's milk protein — the preferred source as in first milks and milks for hungrier babies.
- Soya protein — in soya milk formula, to be used where a vegan diet is being followed and/or where the baby has galactosemia.
- Partially digested (hydrolysed) protein — used in Cow & Gate Comfort, SMA Comfort and Aptamil Comfort, it may help babies with colic or reflux or constipation.

new standards for infant formula

In 2005, for the first time, global consensus was reached by an International Expert Group on infant formula composition. The new recommendations aim to ensure the best possible nutrition for bottle-fed babies, leading to optimal growth, development and future health.

infant formula milks available on the Irish market	
First milks (labelled 'from birth')	Aptamil First or Profutura First Milk Cow & Gate First Infant Milk SMA PRO First Infant Milk
Second milks (from birth, labelled 'for the hungrier baby')	Aptamil Hungry Milk Cow & Gate Infant Milk for Hungrier Babies SMA Extra Hungry Infant Milk
Modified formula for infant feeding problems (from birth)	Aptamil Comfort Cow & Gate Comfort SMA Comfort
Follow-on milks (from 6 months)	Aptamil Follow On or Profutura Follow-On Milk Cow & Gate Follow-on Milk SMA PRO Follow-On-Milk
Soya milks (from birth)	SMA Wysoy

choose cow's milk-based formula

Cow's milk-based infant formula should be the first choice for feeding healthy babies who are not exclusively breastfed. First milks — cow's milk-based infant formula — provide the closest match to breast milk and should always be the first choice for your baby. Examples include Aptamil First or Profutra First Milk, Cow & Gate First Infant Milk, and SMA PRO First Infant Milk.

Optional extra ingredients in formula

The composition of infant formula is very strictly regulated as to its minimum and maximum nutrient content. Manufacturers are allowed, but not obliged, to add a number of extra ingredients. The three main optional ingredients are nucleotides, long chain polyunsaturates (LCPs), and prebiotics.

In 2014 the European Food Safety Authority Panel on Dietetic Products, Nutrition and Allergies reviewed the available research on the beneficial effects for the baby of adding these ingredients to infant formula. With the exception of the long chain polyunsaturate DHA, the panel advised that there is currently insufficient evidence to recommend the routine addition of nucleotides and prebiotics to infant formula. While the addition of these ingredients is not harmful, clear benefits have not been shown and more research is needed.

Long chain polyunsaturates (LCPs) include docosahexaenoic acid (DHA), more commonly known as an omega-3 fat or fish oil, and arachidonic acid (AA) which belongs to the omega-6 family. DHA is an important component of eye, brain and nerve cells and is involved in normal brain and visual development. The developing brain accumulates large amounts of DHA during the first two years of life. LCPs are commonly found in foods such as meat and oily fish. They are naturally present in breast milk. (See Chapter 1, page 10 for more on DHA and AA.)

Prebiotics are food for 'good bacteria'. Prebiotics are not digested in the small bowel but reach the large bowel where they stimulate (promote) the growth of good bacteria. There are over 200 different prebiotics (or oligosaccharides) in breast milk which help block harmful bacteria from attaching to the wall of the baby's gut. They are also thought to boost immunity levels.

It is impossible to achieve the same type and levels of prebiotics in infant formula, or to mimic the various ways they interact with the baby's gut. While the addition of prebiotics to infant formula is not harmful, more research is required on their benefits.

Soya infant formula

Soya infant formula is specially adapted to meet the nutritional needs of the growing baby. It was first introduced in 1929 for infants with cow's milk allergy. However, it is no longer the first choice for an infant with cow's milk allergy, especially those less than 6 months old. This is because we now know that soya protein itself can cause a variety of allergic reactions and that 10–40 per cent of babies with cow's milk allergy are also allergic to soya. Not only is it possible to acquire an allergy to soya but also some scientists believe there may be a link between soya protein and the development of peanut allergy.

Concerns regarding the long-term health effects of soya protein

Soya is a plant protein and contains a group of substances similar to the hormone oestrogen but much weaker in effect. The scientific name for this group of substances is phyto-oestrogens. Scientists have suggested that the consumption of phyto-oestrogens could affect a baby's hormone levels and developing hormonal system. Small babies or babies less than 6 months old on soya-based formula are most at risk as they have the highest intake of formula relative to their body size.

A study published in the *Journal of the American Medical Association* in 2001 showed that women fed on soya formula as infants had slightly longer periods and experienced slightly greater discomfort during menstruation than women who were fed cow's milk formula. However, no other ill effects in either men or women were reported. Medical research trials are ongoing in this area but to date there is no evidence of any serious adverse consequences of soya formula intake on adult sexual and reproductive health.

Until results from further medical research trials become available, it is as well to avoid soya formula in most cases for infants less than 6 months old where a safe and acceptable alternative is available. However, there are important exceptions.

don't give solids too soon
Solids should never be added to the bottle nor should they be introduced in spoon feeds before 4 months (17 weeks) of age.

babies' amazing rate of growth
During the first year of life a healthy baby doubles in length and trebles in weight. By the age of 2 years the baby's brain has grown to 80 per cent of adult size. To support this rapid growth babies have very high nutrient requirements.

The Department of Health and Children
recommends that infants who are not being breastfed should be given a whey-dominant formula until they are 12 months old when cow's milk can be introduced.

it's best not to switch formulas too often

If your baby is having minor feeding difficulties you should always speak to your health professional before making any changes to feeds. It can be very easy to fall into the trap of playing 'milk roulette', switching from one formula to another, but this is very unsettling for babies.

first milk, which best resembles breast milk, should be the formula of choice for most babies. There is no need to change to any other formula — your baby can drink first milk until starting on cow's milk at about 1 year old.

if your baby has colic or reflux

For advice on which formula to use if your baby has colic or reflux and on common infant feeding problems, see Chapter 7.

lactose

Unlike soya-based infant formula, breast milk and all cow's-milk-based infant formulas contain lactose.

Soya milk formula should be given to

- Babies of vegan mothers who do not breastfeed.
- Babies with the medical condition galactosemia.
- Babies with cow's milk protein allergy who refuse to take an extensively hydrolysed formula such as Aptamil Pepti or Nutramigen. For more on cow's milk allergy see Chapter 8.

In these three situations the risks associated with not giving a soya based infant formula are far greater than any potential negative effects phyto-oestrogens may have on long-term health.

Protein and glucose syrup in soya formula

The soya-based SMA Wsoy adheres to EU guidelines on type and level of soya protein. Soya protein is less digestible and of slightly lower quality than cow's milk protein so this formula has a higher protein content than cow's milk formulae. This ensures that babies receiving soya formula obtain sufficient protein for normal growth and development. SMA Wysoy contains DHA and nucleotides.

Glucose syrup is used in soya formulas as a replacement for lactose, the naturally occurring sugar in breast milk and cow's milk-based formula. It is completely safe for babies and is a necessary addition to soy formula.

Since tooth decay can be caused by prolonged contact of glucose syrup with teeth it is best to discourage sucking at a bottle for prolonged periods. It is a good idea to start offering drinks from a beaker from 6 months of age. Once the first teeth have appeared good dental hygiene practices are essential.

Goat's milk

In 2012 the European Food Safety Authority Panel on Dietetic Products, Nutrition and Allergies conducted a detailed review of the suitability of goat's milk protein as a source of protein in infant formula and in follow-on formula. The panel concluded that protein from goat's milk can be suitable as a protein source for infant and follow-on formula provided the final composition complies with EU Infant Formula Compositional Guidelines. Similar to cow's milk, the protein and mineral content of goat's milk is too high for babies and the levels of the amino acids tryptophan and cysteine too low. Just like cow's milk, goat's milk requires modification to make it suitable for babies. Since

March 2014 goat's milk based infant formula is allowed to be sold within the EU. Nanny Care First Infant Milk is available to purchase in Ireland. At the present time this formula does not contain the long chain polyunsaturate DHA (see optional ingredients page 46).

Goat's milk should never be given to a baby with a cow's milk allergy because cow's milk protein and goat's milk protein are very similar and it is highly likely that a cross-reaction will occur—a baby who has an allergy to cow's milk is very likely to be allergic to goat's milk as well.

formula regulations

The manufacture and composition of all infant formula is strictly regulated. Manufacturers have to comply with EU Guidelines which are enforced in all member states. These guidelines dictate the minimum and maximum amount of every nutrient present in the formula as well as the quality of ingredients used.

breast or first milk and a good weaning diet will meet your baby's nutritional needs

It is natural during the first year of life, when so many milestones are being passed, to wish to see your baby's diet progress. Formula milk manufacturers are aware of this and offer a range of products targeted at the different developmental stages of the first three years of life.

The World Health Organisation advocates breast milk from birth up to 2 years of age and beyond (most children stop breastfeeding by the time they are 3 years old). Unlike the many different infant formulas available, the nutrient content of breast milk does not change significantly over this time.

If your baby is eating suitable weaning foods from 6 months on and drinking 500–600 ml (17–20 fl oz) of a first milk infant formula each day, there is no need to change from this formula as all your baby's nutritional requirements are being met.

Other milks

All bottle-fed babies under 1 year of age should receive an infant formula as their main drink. Other milks, such as oat milk, almond milk etc., cannot meet the nutritional needs of the growing baby who may suffer from malnutrition if given these milks instead of infant formula.

follow-on milks

contain up to twice as much iron as first milks and milks for hungrier babies. They also contain more calcium and phosphorus than standard infant formula.

Toddler Milks/Growing-up Milks

Toddler milks are the latest addition to the range of formulas available to parents. They are a type of infant formula made suitable for older children and marketed as an alternative to cow's milk for babies from the age of 12 months. They have

soya milk

Unmodified soya milk is not suitable for babies because of its high protein, low calorie and high sodium (salt) content — up to 3 times higher than in breast milk. A baby's immature kidneys can't cope with such high levels of protein and sodium.

goat's milk

Like unmodified cow's milk and unmodified soya milk, fresh goat's milk is completely unsuitable for babies under 1 year of age. It does not offer a single extra health benefit over cow's milk.

added iron and other vitamins and minerals. Some brands also contain prebiotics. You can find them in the supermarket close to the infant formula and baby foods.

While toddler milks do provide vitamins and minerals, it is far better for your child to get these nutrients from a variety of solid foods. Your toddler needs to learn to eat a range of different foods that will provide the nutrients needed throughout childhood and adulthood. If you rely on toddler milk, problems may arise when your child decides not to drink the milk any more, whereas a child eating a range of different foods who decides to dislike one type can usually obtain similar nutrients from another food. It is important to expose your child while young to a range of foods to help broaden the taste buds.

However, if your child is a very resistant eater and you are worried about his or her intake of iron and other vitamins and minerals, the toddler milks may be a useful source of extra nutrients while you work on increasing the variety of foods your child will eat.

Preparing bottle feeds

5

There is a very wide range of bottles and teats available, so choosing which ones to buy can be difficult. No one brand offers significant advantages over another but the information in this chapter on the brands available will help you in your choice.

Good hygiene practices are essential for safe preparation of bottle feeds. Whether you are giving your baby infant formula or expressed breast milk you need to sterilise all feeding equipment until your baby is 12 months old. In this chapter we look at the different methods of sterilising feeding equipment and advise how to make up and store infant formula in the safest way.

As it is natural for you as a parent to want to check your baby's feed intake we also give information on normal feeding patterns and a guide to how much formula your baby should drink in a day.

Choosing bottles and teats

Brands available on the Irish market include Avent, Dr Brown, Nuk, Tommee Tippee and own brands such as Boots, Mothercare and Tesco. You may notice that many if not all brands claim to provide the closest match to the breastfeeding experience. However, bottle-feeding is completely different to breastfeeding and no one brand is superior to another. Which brand to choose is simply a matter of personal choice, both yours and your baby's. Easy availability, durability and cost are three factors worth considering.

Bottles

Bottles come in two basic shapes—standard neck and wide neck. Wide neck is the newer model of babies' bottle and may make feed preparation and cleaning a little easier, although these bottles do take up more room in the steriliser unit and require slightly more storage space.

When buying bottles check that they are compatible with any other feeding equipment you may already have and want to use e.g. sterilisers.

Bottles are usually available in two sizes—smaller bottles with a 120–150 ml capacity and bigger bottles with a 240–300 ml capacity. From as early as 2 months of age a baby may take more than 150 mls (5 oz) at a feed.

Some bottles, such as Dr Brown's and Tommee Tippee Anti-Colic Plus bottles, have a special vent inside which helps to eliminate air bubbles during a feed and may help reduce wind and colic. These bottles can be more expensive and are a little bit more difficult to clean.

Teat flow rates

Teats are available for both wide neck and standard neck bottles and come in a range of flow rates. Wide neck teats have a broader base and are marketed as having a more 'breast like' or 'easy latch-on' shape.

Flow rates of teats depend on the size or number of holes in the teat and can be broadly categorised into slow, medium and fast. It is also possible to buy variable flow teats where the flow rate of the individual teat can be varied.

The baby's age and type of formula are the two main factors determining which flow rate is suitable. For instance, new-born babies or babies being offered breast milk will usually need a slow flow teat.

Bottles usually come with a slow flow teat as standard and a full range of teats is sold separately. Detailed information regarding flow rates can be found on the packaging.

Avent, Nuk, Tommee Tippee and Dr Brown recommend that only their teats should be used with their bottles. Boots, Mothercare and Tescos wide neck teats should fit most wide neck bottles and their standard neck teats should fit standard bottles.

The different flow rates are usually recommended as suitable for babies of a particular age but this should be regarded as a guide only. It is important that the rate of flow suits the baby. Sometimes a change in formula may necessitate a change in teat e.g. thicker formulas such as Cow & Gate Comfort or Aptamil Comfort may not flow adequately through a slow flow teat.

Anti-colic valves

Many teats now have an in-built anti-colic valve, e.g. the Nuk Air System, Avent Airflex Valve or Tommee Tippee Easi-vent, which work by reducing the negative pressure created in the bottle when a baby sucks on the teat. This decreases the amount of air the baby swallows while feeding and may help reduce wind and colic. The teats don't collapse during a feed and therefore don't have to be periodically removed from the baby's mouth.

Orthodontic shape

These teats have a special shape and are marketed as helping to encourage the baby's correct oral development.

Silicone or latex?

The teats available are made in either silicone or latex. Which type you use is a matter of personal choice and indeed babies sometimes prefer one to the other.

your baby's preferences

As a parent you will learn about your baby's preferences, though this may take a little time. Close observation of your baby during feeding will help you decide whether a particular teat is suitable or not. If your baby is a poor feeder a change of bottle and/or teat may help.

rate of flow of milk

If the milk flow is too slow or too fast, the baby may swallow air while feeding and this will cause wind. Signs to watch out for include too rapid swallowing, milk leaking from the baby's mouth or very hard sucking by the baby.

Teats made from latex have a smooth, skin-like texture and if a breastfed baby refuses to drink from a bottle, trying a latex teat may help. The hole in a latex teat can be made bigger if necessary. It is not safe to do this with silicone teats as they are more likely to tear and bits could break off into your baby's mouth.

Silicone teats are transparent in colour while latex teats are semi-opaque yellow/brown in colour.

How to make the hole in a latex teat bigger

With a sterile, pointed nail scissors cut down into the teat hole making a small incision. Remember, the older the baby the stronger the suck; if the hole is made too big the baby may suck too much formula.

There is no easy way to check if the new size of the hole suits your baby without giving some formula to drink. You will know by watching your baby if the re-sized teat suits. Widen just one teat to begin with until you're sure the new size suits your baby.

Cleaning and sterilising feed equipment

All bottle-feeding equipment (bottles, teats, lids) and any utensils (e.g. knife, whisk) used during the mixing of the feed should be thoroughly cleaned and then sterilised until your baby is 12 months old. This is to ensure that any harmful bacteria are removed to prevent them from growing and multiplying in the feed and making your baby ill.

Teats and bottles should be checked regularly for signs of wear and damage. If you are unsure about the condition of a bottle or teat, it's safer to throw it away.

Before handling any sterile items it is essential to wash your hands with hot soapy water and dry them with a fresh cloth or disposable paper towels. Hand-washing reduces the number of bacteria on the skin but does not get rid of them completely. For this reason, once equipment has been sterilised take great care not to touch the inside of bottles, sealing discs, caps etc. Ideally, use a sterile tongs to handle teats.

Teats and caps should not be placed directly onto work surfaces and once bottles are assembled the cap should always be fitted tightly in place.

Cleaning

You should use hot water with washing-up liquid to clean feeding equipment. Scrub the inside and outside of bottles with a bottle brush. Wash teats inside out or use a teat brush and pay particular attention to the rim and screw top of the bottle.

Try to wash bottles and teats straight away after a feed or at the very minimum rinse them in warm tap water immediately after use. Bacteria can multiply very quickly in any remaining milk and form a film on the bottle which can be very difficult to wash away. After rinsing, the bottles can be left to one side until you are ready to wash them.

It is important to remove all traces of feed from every piece of equipment as feed residue is a perfect breeding ground for bacteria and sterilising equipment may be ineffective if all traces of formula have not been removed during cleaning.

Ideally you should keep any utensils that you use to prepare your baby's feeds separate from the others and use them only for this purpose. Plastic utensils tend to be more durable and, unlike stainless steel, they can be sterilised using a chemical solution such as Milton or in a microwave steam steriliser (provided the plastic is microwave proof).

Bottle and teat brushes don't need to be sterilised but should be stored in a clean place.

Dishwashers can be used to clean equipment provided the equipment is dishwasher proof but dishwashers do not sterilise equipment. Follow the manufacturer's instructions on the stacking of the bottles, caps etc. and inspect the items after the wash to make sure that they are completely clean.

If you hand wash equipment be sure to rinse it thoroughly before sterilising.

Methods of sterilising

The main methods used for sterilising feed equipment are:

- Steam sterilising
- Cold water chemical sterilising e.g. Milton
- Boiling
- Microwaving

Steam sterilising This is the best method. Both electric and microwave steam sterilisers are available. When buying a steriliser check whether it is compatible with any feeding equipment you want to use or have already.

Bags for sterilising equipment in the microwave are also available e.g. Lindam microwave steriliser bags. They work on the same principle as a microwave steam steriliser and may be convenient when travelling (provided a microwave is readily available).

Once the bottle feeding equipment has been thoroughly cleaned and rinsed it should be placed in the steriliser according to the manufacturer's instructions. The length of time required varies, but equipment is usually sterilised in less than 10 minutes. Sterilisers also vary as to how long equipment remains sterile inside them. It's best to sterilise equipment just before you need it.

hygiene
Babies' immune systems are immature and for this reason they are very susceptible to infections from bacteria and viruses. Milk is the perfect medium for bacteria to grow and multiply. Good hygiene is important to protect your baby from infection, particularly tummy bugs (gastroenteritis).

Cold water chemical sterilising Milton is probably the best-known cold water chemical steriliser but there are other products available. They come in tablet or liquid forms. The sterilising solution should be made up according to the manufacturer's instructions. Special containers are available but any non-metallic container can be used to hold the solution e.g. a plastic bowl or ice-cream container.

Clean all the utensils thoroughly in hot water with washing up liquid and rinse them before placing them in the sterilising solution.

When placing bottles, teats etc. in the sterilising solution, make sure no air bubbles are trapped inside. All the surfaces of the feeding equipment need to be in contact with the sterilising liquid. Slowly lower the bottles into the container so that they fill up with the solution. A floating cover (or a plate) should be placed over equipment to make sure that everything remains under the water. Items are generally ready for use after 15–30 minutes—check the manufacturer's instructions. It is safe to leave items in the solution until you need them, for up to a maximum of 24 hours. After 24 hours a fresh solution should be prepared.

Ideally, items should only be removed from the sterilisng solution as they are needed. There is no need to rinse them, simply shake off excess fluid. However, if you do choose to rinse items, you must use cooled boiled water.

Cold water sterilising can be useful if you only need to sterilise a small number of items or when travelling. It is not the most environmentally friendly method, being toxic to aquatic organisms.

Disposable cold water sterilising bags which come with their own sterilising tablets (e.g. Oasis Steriliser Bags, available in Boots) can be used to sterilise feeding equipment using a cold water chemical solution. The bags hold the sterilising solution and feeding equipment. This might be useful when travelling away from home.

Boiling To sterilise by boiling, add feeding equipment to a pan full of cold water. Make sure that all items are fully covered with water and that no air bubbles are trapped inside bottles, teats, etc.

clean hands
You should always wash your hands in hot soapy water before handling feeding equipment or after changing your baby's nappy. If it is not possible to wash your hands, anti-septic wipes or an anti-bacterial hand gel could be used instead.

Cover the pan with a tight-fitting lid, bring to the boil and boil for at least 3 minutes, making sure the pan does not boil dry. The pan should then be kept covered until the feeding equipment is needed. Keep this saucepan for sterilising equipment only.

While boiling water can be used to sterilise all feeding equipment, certain items, especially teats, tend to wear out faster using this method.

Microwaving Some bottles, e.g. Mothercare 'Steriliser' bottles, can be sterilised in the microwave. No additional equipment is necessary. The sterilising takes about 1½ minutes.

Pre-sterilised ready-to-use disposable bottles and teats These bottles, e.g. 'steri-bottle', come individually wrapped and can be used straight away. They can only be used once but the plastic can be recycled. The range includes a 0–3 month bottle and a 3-month plus bottle.

removing feed equipment from the steriliser

It is best to sterilise feeding equipment just before it is needed. If you need to sterilise equipment in advance of preparing feeds, check the manufacturer's instructions on how long it is safe to leave equipment in the steriliser.

If you remove equipment from the steriliser but can't use it straight away, you should cover and store it in a clean, dry place. Assemble feeding bottles thoroughly with the teat pointing down into the bottle and the protective disk in place or with the teat in the position ready for feeding with the cap firmly in place to prevent contamination of the inside of the bottle and the inside and outside of the teat. Bottle caps and discs should fit tightly over the teat so that the outside of the teat remains sterile. Once assembled correctly bottles will remain sterile for 24 hours.

Making up bottle feeds

Before starting to make up bottles you should thoroughly clean the work surfaces and thoroughly wash your hands in hot soapy water. Then boil the water for the feed and allow it to cool for 30 minutes but no longer.

What water should be used to make up infant formula?

It is essential to use freshly boiled tap water to make up infant formula. Empty the kettle, run the cold tap for a few seconds and then fill the kettle. Don't boil the kettle more than once because this may increase the concentration of certain minerals.

Artificially softened water from a fitted water softener is not suitable for the preparation of infant formula due to its high salt content. When fitting a water softener a drinking tap supplying non-softened water should always be retained.

If tap water is unsuitable or unsafe e.g. if you are on holidays abroad or there is a problem with your water supply, you may need to use bottled water. Many natural mineral and spring waters are unsuitable for making up infant formula due to the presence of high levels of sodium (salt) and minerals. Sparkling or fizzy water should never be used. You will need to select a still water with a sodium content of less than 200 mg per 1000 mls/1 litre by checking the nutritional label on the bottle.

Avoid bottled waters containing concentrations of sulphate higher than 250mg/L.

Bottled water for infant formula preparation must always be boiled. Do not boil water more than once. Some bottled waters state on the label if they are suitable for preparation of infant feeds. It is still a good idea to double check the sodium and sulphate content.

guidelines on the safe preparation of powdered infant formula

Infant formula powder is not a sterile product. It can contain harmful bacteria such as cronobacter or salmonella. Infections caused by these bacteria in formula milk are very rare but when they do happen they can be fatal. Cronobacter species is a cause of meningitis. Premature and low birth weight babies, babies whose immunity is compromised and all babies under 2 months old are most at risk.

The bacteria cannot be destroyed during the manufacturing process, but are destroyed by making up the formula using water at a temperature of 70°C. Boiling water has a temperature of 100°C. Once water has reached boiling point, it should be left to cool to 70°C which will take 30 minutes but no longer. Using water hotter than 70°C will cause excessive loss of certain vitamins.

(Food Safety Authority of Ireland 2012)

Boil the water and allow it to cool

If you use an electric kettle to boil water for formula, always allow the kettle to switch itself off. Boil at least one litre of water. Boiling water should be left to cool in the kettle with the lid in place. It is important to leave the water to cool for 30 minutes but no longer. In this way, the water remains hot enough to destroy the bacteria present in the formula powder but not the essential nutrients.

Add the powder to the boiled water

Having boiled the water and allowed it to cool for 30 minutes but no longer you are ready to prepare the feed. Pour the required amount of hot boiled water into a sterile bottle. Always pour the water in first. Add the infant formula powder following the manufacturer's instructions using the scoop provided. Level the powder off with a sterile knife—don't press down on the powder. Re-assemble the bottle tightly and carefully. Shake or swirl well to mix the powder with the water until it is fully dissolved.

Note It is possible that steam from the hot water could wet the powder in the scoop, preventing accurate dosage by causing powder to stick to the scoop. A damp scoop should not be re-inserted into the dry powder in the tin, as it could cause the powder to become moist and allow bacterial growth. If powder sticking on the scoop is a problem, formula could be measured into a clean, sterile, dry container and then added to the water in one go.

making feeds up to the right concentration

Over- or under-concentrating feeds can be harmful to your baby's health and wellbeing. To prepare feeds at the correct concentration the previously boiled water should always be poured into the bottle first. Check that the water level is correct before adding the milk powder.

Fill the scoop provided in the tin with powder and level it off using a sterile knife. Don't use more or less than this amount or you will make your baby ill.

When making up infant formula always use the scoop provided in the actual tin as different products have different scoop sizes, or the scoop for a particular product may change. In Ireland and the UK the standard measure for all infant formula is 1 scoop of formula powder to 30 ml or 1 fl oz of water. This may not be the case in other countries. If buying formula abroad, always check the instructions on the tin when making up feeds.

Never compress the powder in the scoop as this can result in dramatic over-concentration of the feeds.

Solids should not be added to your baby's bottle as this may result in excessive weight gain and/or potentially delay progress onto solid foods. Spoon feeds are important for a baby's development. (See Chapter 6 for more detailed information on when to start solids.)

Note During feed preparation take care to avoid scalding yourself.

Formula Preparation Machines

Formula preparation machines are relatively new to the Irish market and are marketed as being a sterile and convenient method of preparing formula feeds at the correct temperature for consumption, within minutes. Neither the Food Safety Authority of Ireland or the Food Standards Agency UK recommend the use of these machines, as there is insufficient data available regarding their safety. The use of cold tap water that has been boiled once and then cooled for 30 minutes but no longer to greater than 70 degrees Celsius remains the safest way to prepare powdered infant formula. For further information visit the website www.firststepsnutrition.org to read their detailed statement on formula preparation machines.

Cooling and storing feeds

Once the bottles of formula have been made up it is important to cool them quickly. Hold the bottle(s) under cold running tap water or sit them in a large volume of cold or iced tap water. Make sure the water does not come into contact with the cap or neck of the bottle as this can draw water into the bottle and contaminate the feed with harmful bacteria. When cooling and storing bottles the cap should always be fitted tightly in place.

vary the temperature
It can be a good idea to slightly vary the temperature of the milk from time to time or your baby may get fussy and refuse the formula unless it is at an exact temperature.

ready-to-feed liquid formula in cartons undergoes a special heat treatment during manufacturing and is sterile. It can be used instead of powdered infant formula if preferred. You still need to sterilise the feeding bottles and teats.

Wipe the bottles dry with a clean cloth. If you do not need to feed your baby immediately place all the bottles in the coolest part of the fridge—see page 34. The temperature of the fridge must not exceed 5°C. Don't place bottles in the door of the fridge. Bottles can be stored in the fridge for up to 24 hours. After this time any unused feed must be discarded.

If you are using a feed immediately after making it up, cool the milk as above and then check its temperature before feeding your baby. Shake the bottle and drip a little milk onto the inside of your wrist. It should feel lukewarm, not hot. If it still feels hot, cool it some more before feeding. Discard any unused feed after 2 hours.

Re-warming refrigerated bottle feeds

Feed should only be removed from the fridge just before you need it. You can warm the feed using a bottle warmer or by simply placing the bottle in a container e.g. a jug of warm water. To prevent contamination always make sure the water level is below the neck or lid of the bottle. Shake or swirl the bottle occasionally to make sure the milk heats evenly.

To prevent the growth of harmful bacteria it is important to re-warm feeds for no longer than 15 minutes. Never warm feeds on a radiator or near a fire as this will create the perfect conditions for bacteria to grow and multiply. Always check the temperature of the feed by shaking the bottle and then testing a few drops on the inside of your wrist; the feed should feel lukewarm, not hot.

Microwaves should not be used to re-warm feeds as the milk may heat unevenly creating 'hot spots' which can easily scald a baby's mouth.

After a feed has been heated it should be used within 2 hours. Any milk left over at the end of the feed should be discarded.

Preparing feeds while travelling

If a feed is needed while travelling the safest option is to use a carton of ready-to-feed liquid formula. Unopened cartons of ready-to-feed formula do not need to be stored in the fridge. When heading out simply bring a sterile bottle and an unopened carton of formula with you. Some babies will drink formula at room temperature and it may not be necessary to warm the ready-to-feed formula before feeding.

You may need a clean sterile scissors to open the carton of formula. Shake the bottle before giving it to the baby.

If it is not possible to give your baby a ready-to-feed liquid formula, add boiled water to one or more sterile bottles. Reassemble the bottles according to the manufacturer's instructions and allow the water to cool. Store the bottles of sterile water in a clean place. Bring the bottles of sterile water along with the can of powdered infant formula with you when travelling. It may be more convenient to buy individual sachets of infant formula powder or alternatively you can measure out the required number of scoops of formula powder into a sterile container with lid. If you need to make up more than one bottle, special milk powder dispensers with multiple compartments are available. Remember to discard any unused bottles of sterile water after 24 hours.

Containers should be washed, sterilised and dried before each use.

> **feeding patterns**
> It is never helpful to apply rigid norms to a baby's feeding pattern. Babies often take more formula at some feeds than others. Your baby will be hungrier some days than others. Remember it is not necessary for your baby always to finish the bottle.

Transporting feeds to the crèche or child minder

Feeds for the crèche will need to be prepared in advance, cooled in the fridge and transported in a cool bag with ice packs. Always label the bottles with the name of your child.

Provided the feeds are cold when placed in the cool bag, they will be maintained at a safe temperature for up to 2 hours. They should be placed in a fridge immediately on arrival at your destination.

Feeding patterns

Bottle-fed babies, like breastfed babies, should be fed on demand. This does not mean that you can't establish a feeding routine for your baby e.g. 3–4 hourly feeds. What it does mean is that your baby should be allowed to decide how much formula to take at each feed, in other words to feed to appetite.

It is normal for your baby to drink more formula at some feeds than at others. Feeding to appetite means that your baby learns to recognise when he or she feels full.

Initially, new-born babies may feed every 2–3 hours (timed from the beginning of one feed to the start of the next) and intervals between feeds can be unpredictable during the first few weeks. It is better to watch the baby for signs of hunger than to watch the clock. These signs include the baby moving around in a restless way or making sucking motions with the lips and tongue. By around 2 months many babies are feeding about every 3–4 hours and some even manage without a night feed. If you are lucky, from around 2 months your baby may start sleeping for 6–7 hours overnight, obtaining all nutrition in 5–6 feeds a day.

The table below shows how much and how often you should expect your baby to feed. The figures are a guide only—it is normal for a baby to vary the amount taken from day to day and even from feed to feed.

typical feed intakes of formula-fed infants			
Age	Feed intervals	Number of feeds in 24 hours	Feed volumes per single feed
1–2 weeks	2–3 hourly	7–10	50–70 ml (2 oz)
2–6 weeks	3–4 hourly	6–7	75–100 ml (3 oz)
2 months	3–4 hourly	5–6	120–180 ml (4–6 oz)
3 months	3–4 hourly	5	180–220 ml (6–7 oz)
6 months*	4 hourly	4–5	210–240 ml (7–8 oz)

*At 4–6 months following the introduction of solids, weaning foods will begin to contribute to your baby's nutrient intake. Over time, as the amount of solids your baby eats increases, the number of formula feeds will reduce.

How much formula should my baby be taking?

For the first 6 months your baby should be taking 150–200 mls of formula per 1 kg (or 70–90 mls per lb). For example, a baby weighing 5 kg should take 750–1000 mls in 24 hours (150/200 mls multiplied by 5). It is normal for some babies to take slightly more than this, some a little less. Provided your baby is contented and growing appropriately for age, then there is nothing to worry about.

What position should my baby be in during a bottle feed?

Your baby should be held in a supportive, semi-upright position which encourages eye contact and bonding. It is good to alternate the side you hold your baby for feeds—if you use your right arm for the first feed use the left arm for the next and so on.

How long should it take my baby to drink a bottle?

About 20 minutes is the right length of time for a feed but some babies are slow feeders and others fast. A slow feed could last up to one hour and a fast feed may be finished in 10 minutes. The flow of milk from the teat and wind are two factors that may affect your baby's feeding. (See Chapter 7 for more information on techniques for winding your baby.)

Does my baby need additional drinks?

Formula will provide a healthy baby with all the fluid needed in the first 6 months of life. It's only when your baby is unwell or very thirsty e.g. during hot weather, that additional drinks are needed. For a thirsty baby, cooled, boiled tap water is the best drink to offer. An unwell baby with diarrhoea needs to be given an oral reyhdration solution (see Chapter 7, pages 114–5).

Weaning and progressing to family meals

6

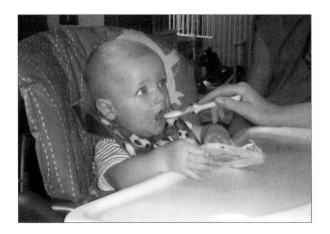

Weaning is a gradual process of introducing solid foods into your baby's diet so that by the age of 12 months he or she is eating family foods and taking part in family mealtimes. The transition can be tricky and yes, it's messy, but also a lot of fun!

There are a lot of misconceptions about what are acceptable weaning foods. This chapter sets out clearly which solid foods you should be giving your baby and at what stage. It will guide you through the process of establishing a varied and nutritious diet for your child.

When should weaning begin?

Weaning should begin when your baby is aged around 6 months. For nutritional and developmental reasons, the introduction of solid food to a baby's diet should not begin before the baby is 4 months (17 weeks) old, nor should it be delayed beyond 6 months (26 weeks).

Breast milk or formula milk provides all the nutrition a baby needs for the first 6 months of life. However, if you feel your baby needs solid food before 6 months ask your public health nurse for advice.

babies should start on solids at around 6 months

The Department of Health and Children (following World Health Organisation recommendations of 2001), advises that all babies should start solids at around 6 months of age. Breast milk or formula milk alone provides adequate nourishment for the first 6 months of a baby's life.

Why weaning should not begin before 4 months (17 weeks)

- The volume of breast and formula milk taken may reduce too soon so that the baby does not achieve essential nutrients.
- The baby's co-ordination may not be developed enough for proper head control to allow sucking and chewing of solid food.
- The baby's gut and kidneys will not be mature enough to cope with solid food.
- There is an increased risk that the baby will develop coeliac disease, Type 1 diabetes or wheat allergy.
- Giving energy-rich foods too soon may result in your baby becoming overweight.

Why weaning should not be delayed beyond 6 months

- A baby's increasing energy and nutrient requirements will not be met by milk alone beyond 6 months of age.
- Older babies may be more difficult to persuade to take solids.
- Babies weaned later are less likely to go on to eat a varied diet.
- Babies weaned later may not advance to family foods until after the first birthday.

Introducing gluten after 7 months of age may increase the risk that the baby will develop coeliac disease, Type 1 diabetes or wheat allergy.

If your baby is born prematurely i.e. more than 3 weeks early, you will need to ask your paediatrician or paediatric dietician when is the best time to introduce solid food. Weaning may be delayed to some time between 5 and 8 months from birth.

The stages of weaning
Weaning takes place in roughly 4 stages, starting with the first spoon feeds when the baby is 4–6 months old and finishing at 12 months. A baby who starts on spoon feeding at 6 rather than 4 months will go through the first two stages more quickly than a younger baby. The sample menus and schedules given later in this chapter should be seen as guidelines only.

How to spoon feed
Changing from sucking for milk to taking food from a spoon is a bewildering experience for babies. It takes a little time for them to learn to take what is to them a strange substance from a spoon and then figure out how to move it from the front of the tongue to the back of the mouth. Your baby may spit and dribble out the food at first and may cry between spoonfuls, having been used to a continual flow of milk from nipple or teat. Remember, infants vary in the length of time it takes them to accept solids. Some will take only a short time whereas others may take several weeks.

When starting spoon feeding
Choose a time of day when both you and your baby are relaxed—spoon feeding should not be hurried.

- Allow plenty of time and enjoy the experience. Go at your baby's pace, don't rush or 'force feed'.
- Be prepared for a mess—have a good supply of dribbling bibs to hand; floor mats or newspapers are also very useful.
- Make sure your baby is well supported in a sitting position, with legs, head, back and feet supported. A car seat is useful to begin with.
- Use a high chair as soon as your baby can manage to sit unsupported.
- Place yourself so that your baby can look straight ahead at you while you are spoon feeding.
- Don't persist if the food is rejected initially, just try again the next day—it will be accepted after a few attempts.

When spoon feeding
Use a small flat spoon and half fill it.
- Rub the spoon gently against the baby's bottom lip, introducing it gently and slowly to the mouth, allowing your baby to suck food from the spoon.
- Place the bowl of the spoon firmly on the centre of the tongue, without pressing, as your baby accepts the spoon. This will keep the baby's jaw and tongue from thrusting forward.
- Give small spoonfuls of food; it's easier for your baby to move a small volume of food around the mouth.
- Avoid lifting the spoon out of the mouth and scraping the food off in doing so. Take it out of the mouth straight; this encourages your baby to use the lips to close around the spoon to take the food.
- Avoid wiping your baby's mouth during spoon feeding. As your baby learns to swallow efficiently drooling decreases.
- Look out for signs of tiredness, don't push your baby to frustration. Infants are learning the skill of eating so it is important to be patient.

What is the best time to give a spoon feed?
Begin by giving a spoon feed once a day, at a time when your baby is relaxed, alert and in good form. Midday or in the afternoon are usually the best times. Offer the spoon at the end or part way through a milk feed, when your baby is not too hungry.

As soon as your baby is managing 5–6 teaspoons at a single spoon feed or mealtime start offering a second spoon feed in the day. Some babies can go faster, others will be slower.

Baby-Led Weaning
Baby-led weaning (BLW) is an approach to introducing solid foods that allows your baby to self-feed from the very start of weaning. Instead of spoon-feeding, parents let their baby 'lead the way' by feeding themselves finger foods whilst joining in at family meals.

Should you choose this approach to weaning your baby, introduce foods around six months of age. Self-feeding is not recommended before six months of age as the vast majority of infants will not be developmentally ready, nor will they have the necessary motor skills. For self-feeding, your baby will need to be able to sit with little or no help and to reach for and pick up food. These skills develop in the majority of infants at six months of age but may not develop until eight months of age in some.

The first foods offered at six months must be soft. Suitable first finger foods include soft-cooked sweet potato, soft-cooked broccoli, ripe avocado slices and slices of soft mozzarella cheese. As discussed later in the chapter (page 73), it is extremely important to introduce iron-rich foods from six months of age.

Foods presenting a choking risk to babies include raw apple and raw or undercooked carrot, and these should be avoided. Round foods such as grapes and cherry tomatoes should always be cut in quarters. Babies should never be left alone while eating.

Babies are growing rapidly, and it is important that their food and nutrient intake meets their nutritional needs. In order to self-feed successfully, babies need to have sufficient physical stamina. There are certain times, e.g. during and following a period of illness, where baby-led weaning may require some modification.

Stage 1 Starting spoon feeds (the first 2 weeks of weaning)

Up until now your baby has had only breast or formula milk. When you begin weaning you are getting your baby used to a spoon, and introducing texture to your baby's mouth, rather than providing any extra nourishment. Don't reduce milk feeds yet. Continue to breastfeed on demand or give your baby the usual amount of infant formula milk.

First foods

The very first foods must be easy to digest. The texture needs to be runny (semi-liquid) and absolutely smooth, similar to runny yogurt in consistency with no lumps.

> **potato purée** is best not tried in the first few weeks. It is difficult to make into a runny purée.

stage 1 (the first 2 weeks)

Milk feed Breastfeed on demand or continue to give the usual volume of formula milk. Don't decrease the volume of milk too quickly.

Number of meals per day 1–2 Approximate size of each meal 1–6 teaspoons.

Texture of food Smooth, runny purée, no lumps.

Cereals Baby rice, ground white rice.

Vegetables Root vegetables: carrots, turnip, parsnip, butternut squash.

Fruit Ripe fruit: uncooked banana; stewed apple and pear.

Meat and meat alternatives Once the baby is accepting food from a spoon: soft, well-cooked meat, poultry, fish (remove all bones); peas, beans and lentils can be puréed then mixed with vegetable.

Cow's milk Small amounts of full-fat cow's milk can be mixed into solids but it's best to use expressed breast milk or formula milk at this stage.

Dairy foods Natural yogurt (full fat).

Suitable first foods

- Baby rice
- Puréed root vegetables: carrot, turnip, parsnip, and butternut squash
- Puréed ripe fruits: banana or stewed apple or pear

savoury before sweet
It is a good idea to introduce savoury purées, such as vegetables, before sweet purées such as fruit, as babies who have got used to sweet foods may be reluctant to accept savoury tastes. Babies have a natural desire for sweet tastes.

Baby rice can be mixed with breast milk, formula milk or cooled boiled water, making it just a little thicker than milk. Babies tend to prefer it when their usual milk is used—expressed breast milk or formula—as they recognise the taste.

Cook vegetables and fruit until tender and soft (some very ripe soft fruit needs no cooking). Liquidise, then pass through a metal sieve with a fork to remove all small lumps and form a smooth texture. Then the formula or expressed breast milk can be added to the purée to make it almost liquid.

Don't add salt or sugar, or put rusk, cereal or other foods into your baby's bottle. (See pages 87–8 for more on preparing baby rice and purées.)

The first months of weaning are a critical period for getting your baby to accept new tastes. Don't be afraid to try lots of different foods – the quicker you introduce new flavours the better. It will take longer for your baby to accept bitter tastes such as broccoli. Don't give up – keep going! As little as ½ a teaspoon a day will eventually induce a preference for that food.

stools may change
When you add solid foods to your baby's diet his or her stools may change colour and odour. This is perfectly normal.

Sample menu for stage 1

Days 1–3 *Early morning* breast/formula *Breakfast* breast/formula *Lunch* breast/formula and 1–2 teaspoons baby rice *Dinner* breast/formula *Bedtime* breast/formula

Days 4–5 *Early morning* breast/formula *Breakfast* breast/formula *Lunch* breast/formula and parsnip purée *Dinner* breast/formula *Bedtime* breast/formula

Day 6 *Early morning* breast/formula *Breakfast* breast/formula *Lunch* breast/formula and parsnip purée with baby rice *Dinner* breast/formula *Bedtime* breast/formula

Day 7 *Early morning* breast/formula *Breakfast* breast/formula *Lunch* breast/formula and pear purée *Dinner* breast/formula *Bedtime* breast/formula

Day 8 *Early morning* breast/formula *Breakfast* breast/formula and pear purée with baby rice *Lunch* breast/formula and parsnip purée with baby rice *Dinner* breast/formula *Bedtime* breast/formula

Days 9–10 *Early morning* breast/formula *Breakfast* breast/formula and pear purée with baby rice *Lunch* breast/formula and carrot purée *Dinner* breast/formula *Bedtime* breast/formula

Days 11–12 *Early morning* breast/formula *Breakfast* breast/formula and banana purée *Lunch* breast/formula and carrot and parsnip purée *Dinner* breast/formula *Bedtime* breast/formula

Day 13 *Early morning* breast/formula *Breakfast* breast/formula and banana purée *Lunch* breast/formula and parsnip and apple *Dinner* breast/formula *Bedtime* breast/formula

Stage 2 Increasing variety and establishing a meal pattern (2 weeks after starting solids)

At this stage you will be establishing a meal pattern for your baby and introducing more flavours. Solids now begin to provide some extra nourishment, especially protein and iron which are so important for your baby's growth and development.

try and try again
Don't expect your baby to accept a new food until it has been offered at least 10 times. You may have to offer it up to 14 or more times before it is accepted.

You can change the consistency of the solid food to a slightly thicker, smooth purée with no lumps.

Continue to breastfeed on demand or give the usual amount of infant formula milk. The breast or formula milk should still supply the main source of nourishment for your baby. During this stage continue to offer solids during or after the milk feed.

Aim for 2–3 meals each day. Then gradually increase the quantity of food at each meal, according to appetite. Be guided by your own and your baby's instincts.

stage 2 (2 weeks after starting spoon feeds)

Milk feed Breastfeed on demand or continue to give the usual volume of formula milk. Don't decrease the volume of milk too quickly.

Number of meals per day 2–3 Approximate size of each meal 5–10 teaspoons.

Texture of food Smooth, slightly thicker purée (add a little less liquid); no lumps.

Cereals Baby rice, ground white rice, baby porridge.

Vegetables Potato and stronger flavoured vegetables: broccoli, spinach, cauliflower, peas, courgettes.

Fruit Peach, plum, kiwi, melon, avocado.

Meat and meat alternatives Once the baby is accepting food from a spoon: soft, well-cooked meat, poultry, fish (remove all bones); peas, beans and lentils can be puréed then mixed with vegetable.

Cow's milk Small amounts of full-fat cow's milk can be mixed into solids but it's best to use expressed breast milk or formula milk at this stage.

Dairy foods Natural yogurt (full fat).

recommendations on allergenic foods

For many years, parents were advised to delay giving their babies any foods that might cause an allergic reaction (allergenic foods). These foods include wheat, dairy products, eggs, fish, nuts, shellfish, soya and citrus fruits. We now know that there is no convincing evidence that these foods should be excluded or introduced late to a baby's diet, even where there is a family history of allergy. Ongoing research in this area suggests delayed introduction of allergenic foods may actually do more harm than good, increasing the risk of food allergy. It is best to introduce potentially allergenic foods one by one, three days apart, so that the baby can be monitored for any adverse reaction to a particular food.

Foods to avoid before the age of 12 months

- Added salt, gravy and sauces.
- Added sugar. It's not necessary and it will encourage a sweet tooth. It may also lead to tooth decay as first teeth start to show.
- Honey is only safe after 12 months as there is a small risk of botulism.
- Soft and unpasteurised cheeses. e.g. blue cheese, brie.
- Cow's milk is not suitable as a drink before the first birthday, but can be taken mixed in with food after 4 months. However, it is better to mix expressed breast milk or formula milk with solids in Stages 1 and 2.
- Hot spices e.g. black pepper, red chilli powder; mild spices such as coriander, cumin and cinnamon can be used sparingly.
- Undercooked eggs. Scrambled and hard-boiled eggs are fine but may be difficult to include in smooth runny purées.
- Nuts: avoid whole or chopped nuts until the age of 5 years due to the risk of choking.
- Liver: contains too much vitamin A for infants.
- Bran: adding bran to your baby's food will reduce their appetite and can impair the absorption of iron, calcium and zinc.
- Predatory fish: shark, marlin, ray and fresh tuna contain high levels of potentially harmful contaminants such as mercury. All other fish, as long as the bones are removed, are safe for infants.
- Processed meats: ham, bacon, sausages and rashers are high in salt and contain additivies which are unsuitable for infants.

When your baby is accepting solids from a spoon, introduce different tastes, including well-cooked puréed meat and pulses. This will expand the range of flavours of your baby's diet and improve the nutritional content. Combine different foods and purée them together, e.g. rice, cauliflower and beef purée.

Meat, poultry and fish (without bones) are very good sources of protein, vitamins and minerals, which your baby needs for growth and development.

Purée well-cooked meat or fish with vegetables and baby rice or potato mixed with your baby's usual milk to adjust the texture. If giving shop-bought meals, use meat and poultry meals that contain at least 2.5 g of protein in 100 g of food.

Oily fish such as salmon, trout, herring, mackerel and sardines are rich sources of omega-3 fats, which are essential for brain and eye development. Aim to offer your baby 30g of oily fish twice per week from 7 months of age.

Puréed pulses, such as lentils, peas and beans, are also good sources of protein, mineral and vitamins.

Butter and fats Once your baby is taking vegetables, you can add a very small amount of butter, polyunsaturated margarine or vegetable oil, for example olive oil. Don't use low-fat spreads as they contain a lot of water.

Desserts Once your baby has been having 3 meals a day for a week or so, you can start to offer a savoury followed by a dessert. Try stewed fruit mixed with custard or baby rice.

When your baby has learned to take food easily from the spoon, try slightly stiffer purées by adding less liquid (breast milk, infant formula, cooled pre-boiled water) or more ingredients to the plate feeds (e.g. potato or baby rice) as by this stage your baby will have developed a strong sucking action.

The thicker purées will teach your baby to move the food from side to side in the mouth. This is one of the skills needed in due course (at approximately 9 months of age) to move food to the gums or teeth at the back of the mouth to gum or chew.

By 6 months of age babies are able to turn their heads freely and they try playing with their food. Give your baby a spoon with a thick handle to grasp while you are spoon feeding with another spoon.

milk
Don't reduce the amount of milk offered, let your baby's appetite be the guide. The volume taken will gradually go down as the amount of food taken at meal times increases.

meat, poultry and fish are good for the brain
As soon as your baby is accepting food from a spoon you can start offering meat, poultry and fish — there is no need to delay. There is good evidence that including meat, both red and white, in the weaning diet helps brain development and function.

learning to like varied food

Introducing new tastes and textures all the way through the weaning process teaches your child to eat a good range of foods, making it easier to achieve a nutritionally balanced diet. Food preference is shaped by repeated experience; in other words we tend to prefer foods we are used to.

Fish, eggs and soya may be introduced at 26 weeks. This will not increase the risk of allergy/eczema

sample menu at the end of stage 2, after 6–8 weeks of weaning

Breakfast
Initially, baby rice or other baby cereal made with breast or formula milk and topped with puréed fruit (1–2 teaspoons) moving on to Weetabix, Ready Brek or porridge mixed well with breast or formula milk (if over 6 months). Breast or bottle feed.

Mid-morning
Breast or bottle feed.

Lunch
Any of the following:
- [ ] baby rice, parsnip and beef purée
- [ ] potato creamed with your baby's usual milk, carrot and lamb purée
- [ ] potato creamed with your baby's usual milk, cauliflower and salmon purée
- [ ] sweet potato creamed with your baby's usual milk, leek and chicken purée
- [ ] rice, cauliflower and beef purée
- [ ] sweet potato, creamed with your baby's usual milk and blended with puréed broccoli and chick peas
- [ ] red lentil, carrot and potato soup.

Drink Cooled boiled water.

Mid afternoon
Breast or bottle feed.

Evening meal
As at lunch time. At this stage your baby needs the equivalent of a second lunch—dessert-type foods e.g. baby custards, fruit compotes, are not adequate.

Drink Cooled boiled water.

Late evening
Breast or bottle feed.

Stage 3 Increasing texture and introducing finger foods (age 6–9 months)

Over the next 2 to 3 months your baby will play with food and try to feed him or herself. You can increase the range of foods offered. Food need no longer be of purée texture but can be minced or mashed with soft lumps. You can introduce a cup or beaker and finger foods such as pieces of toast and banana. Continue to breastfeed on demand or give infant milk, between 500 and 600 mls (17–20oz) daily.

stage 3 (6–9 months)

Milk feed Breastfeed on demand or give a minimum of 500–600 mls (17-20 oz) of formula milk per day.

Number of meals per day 3. Approximate size of each meal 2–4 tablespoons.

Texture of food Minced and mashed with soft lumps. Introduce soft finger foods.

Cereals Pasta, bread, Weetabix, Ready Brek, porridge, wholemeal bread, rusk; limit foods made with white refined flour e.g. biscuits, cakes.

Vegetables Potato and stronger flavoured vegetables: broccoli, spinach, cauliflower, peas, courgettes; plus leek, onion, cabbage, spinach, sweet corn, tomato, peppers, mushrooms.

Fruit Citrus fruits: remove pith and seed; berry fruits: put through a metal sieve to remove pips and seeds; mango, grapes: peel and deseed, (avoid whole grapes); stewed dried fruit: apricots.

Meat and meat alternatives Soft cooked minced or puréed meat/poultry, fish (remove all bones) or pulses; hard-boiled or scrambled eggs (avoid lightly cooked eggs for young children).

Cow's milk Small amounts of full-fat cow's milk can be mixed into solids or cereal; not to be given as a drink until 12 months old.

Dairy foods Full-fat yogurts; mild hard cheeses; cream.

Foods that may be added to your baby's diet during stage 3

- Cheese and yogurt. Lots of yogurts are marketed at children, but regular yogurts are perfectly suitable and may contain less sugar.
- Pasteurised cow's milk can be used in small amounts in foods.
- Citrus fruits.
- Unsalted nut butters (avoid whole or chopped nuts before the age of 5 years).
- Note: It is safest to boil freshly drawn tap water, which is to be offered as a drink to babies up until 12 months of age.

iron and the weaning diet

- The iron store that your baby is born with is almost depleted at 6 months of age so it is extremely important that the weaning diet includes enough iron-containing foods to promote growth and prevent iron-deficiency anaemia. Small children are more at risk of becoming anaemic than adults because of the extra iron needed for growth. A study on anaemia in children in Ireland found that 1 in 10 two-year-olds were anaemic.
- Red meat, which includes beef, lamb, mutton, pork, is the best source of iron you can offer. Introduce smooth puréed meats into the early weaning diet then coarsely puréed meat and finely chopped meats as you go through the weaning process. Aim to give your child red meat at least 3 times a week.
- Other useful iron-rich foods are eggs, beans, cereals with added iron and dark green vegetables.

Breast milk or infant formula should still be contributing most of your baby's nourishment but as he or she eats more solid food, you can expect the amount of milk taken to reduce. Aim for at least 500–600 mls (17–20 oz) per day. Try to follow your baby's appetite and pace.

As soon as your baby is happily having 3 spoon feeds a day and taking a wider variety of foods, start spacing spoon feeds and milk feeds apart. Aim for 3 or 4 milk feeds a day e.g. early morning, mid morning, mid afternoon and at bedtime, with solids at breakfast, lunch and the evening meal.

Mashed food

When your baby is close to sitting up unaided, playing with food and is putting his or her fingers into the mouth, it's time to start offering thicker and lumpier food.

Mash half the usual meal with a fork and purée the other half, then mix the two together. The texture becomes slightly thicker and lumpier than before. Gradually increase the mashed portion until the meal is completely mashed.

You can also offer soft lumps within foods such as mashed ripe banana or avocado, mashed baked beans, mashed peas, rice pudding. Try to make lumps the same size and softness.

Increasing the texture will encourage a chewing motion. Teeth are not required to handle soft lumps—babies tend to gum things quite effectively. It is much more difficult for babies to accept lumps after the age of 9 months so do keep trying if your baby doesn't take to lumps straight away.

Your baby may cough, gag or heave a little when first offered mashed food; this is normal for many babies starting lumps. It's a reflex reaction that often happens when the new texture or soft lump hits the back of a baby's throat. Stay calm, your baby may panic if you panic, and find it more difficult to swallow the lumpier texture.

Avoid the following lumpy foods initially:

- Some shop-bought stage 2 baby foods (dried or in jars) contain very hard lumps amidst a smooth purée. Your baby may expect a smooth purée then get a shock when lumps are encountered.
- Lumpy cereal with milk e.g. Rice Krispies. The combination of a runny liquid with a lump can be very difficult for your baby to manage at this young age.

---

phasic bite reflex

Once your baby is managing thickened purées he or she will develop a rhythmic bite and release pattern called a phasic bite reflex. The baby seems to be opening and closing the mouth when something touches the gums.

starting solids close to 6 months of age

Begin as outlined in stages 1 and 2. Your baby will be able to go through the early stages quite quickly to the mashed, lumpy and finger foods of stage 3, as coordination is more developed at 6 months.

chewing or gumming

is really important for the development of muscles that your child will use for speech when older. This is one of the reasons babies need to start taking solids from the age of 6 months.

■ Mashed potato can form lumps, which can be difficult for your baby to manage during the early stages of weaning.

Self-feeding

When your baby shows an interest in touching food, it is vital to allow him or her to play with it and explore it; your baby will feel more secure with foods as a result and be more willing to put the food into the mouth. While mealtimes will become much messier and take longer, try and go with it, it's the best way for babies to learn and it is an important step towards independence.

Finger foods

Between 7 and 9 months your baby will begin to pick up objects with the thumb and forefinger; this is known as the pincer grasp, it allows babies to handle and try finger foods for themselves.

The following are ideal first finger foods as they can be easily gummed and digested.

■ Cooked soft vegetables, e.g. carrot, parsnip. Cut into narrow batons.
■ Ripe, peeled fruit, e.g. pear, banana, peach halves or quarters, (not slices).
■ Fingers of buttered toast (no crusts), bread sticks, rice cakes.
■ Long, thin strips of cheese.
■ Well-cooked pasta shapes.
■ Coarsely puréed meats.

Avoid sweet biscuits and rusks so that your baby doesn't get into the habit of expecting sweet snacks.

> **teeth** are not essential for good nutrition during weaning as babies use their gums to chew lumpier food. Whether or not a baby has teeth has no bearing on the weaning process.

Flavours

The more flavours that are experienced at this early stage the less fussy your baby is likely to be later on. A child's preference for certain foods is related to the frequency of exposure to those foods and tastes. So keep trying over and over again.

It is important to include savoury foods, as the taste for sweet foods tends to develop first (this may be due to the exposure to breast milk or formula which contains the natural sugar lactose). You don't want the desire for sweet foods to dominate all other foods and flavours. Potentially it can lead to a limited palate for flavour and an unvaried diet or fussy eating. So try to offer a range of different flavours and tastes: savoury (e.g. meat), bitter (e.g. green vegetables), sour (e.g. natural yogurt) and sweet (e.g. mandarin, carrot).

> **the danger of choking**
> A crawling baby should not be handed finger foods as this can result in choking. Never leave your baby alone when eating in case of choking.

sample menu for the end of stage 3 (age 9 months)

Breakfast
Any of the following:
- unsweetened breakfast cereal e.g. Weetabix, Ready Brek
- porridge with breast milk, formula or whole cow's milk
- mashed fruit mixed with yogurt, fingers of bread/toast with butter or margarine

Drink small amount of freshly drawn tap water from a cup

Mid-morning
Breast or bottle feed

Lunch (or light meal)
Any of the following:
- sandwiches filled with tuna, chopped chicken or ham (cut into small squares)
- pasta shapes in tomato sauce with grated cheese
- scrambled egg with fingers of toast
- homemade soup (liquidised) with a small sandwich
- cheese or baked beans on fingers of toast

Drink small amount of freshly drawn tap water from a cup

Mid-afternoon
Breast or bottle feed

Dinner (or main meal)
Any of the following:
- minced or chopped meat, mashed potatoes and turnip
- chicken casserole and rice
- vegetable risotto and grated cheese
- home-made beef or lentil burgers, tomato slices and boiled potato
- cauliflower cheese and boiled potatoes
- spaghetti bolognese with pasta shapes

Drink small amount of freshly drawn tap water from a cup

Dessert
Any of the following:
- soft fresh fruit quarters, e.g. banana, pear, melon (no seeds)
- tinned soft fruit in natural juice, e.g. pear, peaches
- semolina or rice pudding with chopped soft fruits
- yogurt or fromage frais (full-fat varieties)

Late evening
Breast or bottle feed

Your baby may reject new flavours initially but be reassured this is a very natural reaction. Keep offering the new flavour or food over a few weeks—up to 14 times. Your child's taste buds will become accustomed to the new flavour and will enjoy it.

Introduce a cup

As the volume of solids increases, your baby will tend to get thirsty. This is the perfect opportunity to introduce a cup. Encourage your baby to drink from a cup from 6 months of age. Give cooled boiled tap water from a trainer cup with meals.

Breastfed babies may drink more readily from a cup than bottle-fed babies. If your baby is reluctant to drink from a cup, you need to persist in bringing it out at every meal time—it will work.

Feeding from a bottle should be discouraged completely after the age of 12 months. The reason is that most drinks other than water contain either natural or added sugar. Using a teat means there is prolonged contact with newly growing teeth increasing the risk of tooth decay. The use of teats can also inhibit speech development.

making faces

When tasting certain flavours babies instinctively make a face expressing distaste. Do continue to offer these flavours — don't be put off by the baby's facial expression but focus on his or her willingness to continue eating the food.

Stage 4 Moving to family meals (age 9–12 months)

Now your baby is ready for further variety in the diet. Continue with 3 main meals and include 1–2 snacks each day. The consistency of the food can change from roughly mashed to chopped. Continue with breast milk (on demand) or bottle feeds, approximately 500–600 mls (17–20 oz) daily.

If your child is managing finger foods or is able to move foods from side to side in the mouth try giving food in bite-sized pieces on his or her own plate at mealtimes. Your child can try picking them up and feeding him or herself and should be encouraged to do so.

stage 4 (9–12 months)

Milk feed Breastfeed on demand or give a minimum of 500–600 mls (17-20 oz) of formula milk per day.

Number of meals per day 3 plus 1–2 snacks. Approximate size of each meal 4–6 table-spoons.

Texture of food Minced and finely chopped; finger foods increase.

Cereals Pasta, bread, Weetabix, Ready Brek, porridge, or other breakfast cereal, wholemeal bread, rusk; limit foods made with white refined flour e.g. biscuits, cakes.

Vegetables Wide range.

Fruit Wide range.

Meat and meat alternatives Increase variety; introduce stronger flavoured fish e.g. oily fish—mackerel, tuna, salmon (remove all bones).

Cow's milk Small amounts of full-fat cow's milk can be mixed into solids or cereal; not to be given as a drink until 12 months old.

Dairy foods Full-fat yogurts; mild hard cheeses; cream.

If by 9 months your baby is having thick purées and has not tried mashed foods, skip that stage and try offering chopped-up foods instead. Most foods served at family meals only need to be minced or chopped and are suitable for your child at this stage e.g. chopped meat and vegetables, or small pasta shapes.

Serve the foods separately, rather than mixed together, on the plate so that, for example, the pieces of potato, vegetable and meat do not touch each other. Your child will then start to visually identify different foods and will also associate the taste with the particular food.

salt in breakfast cereal

A common misconception is that regular breakfast cereals are too high in salt for infants. This is not generally the case e.g. one biscuit of Weetabix contains 0.05 g salt. (Remember to check nutrition labels.) A limit of 1 g of salt a day is recommended for babies between 6 and 12 months old.

fat

1 g of fat produces almost 10 calories, making it extremely energy dense. A lot of calories can be obtained from a small serving.

avoid added salt

When cooking for the family take out a portion before seasoning so your baby can share the family meals. Avoid foods that contain a lot of salt, e.g. stock cubes, packet soups and sauces, crisps, bacon, smoked meats.

Salt

As your child eats more adult foods, so the intake of salt may also increase. You can limit the intake of salt in various ways: by cutting down on packet and processed foods, which are very high in salt, e.g. tinned spaghetti, chicken nuggets. It is best not to add salt to cooking water for vegetables or to food before serving it. It's good for the whole family to keep salt intake down.

Offer a variety of foods from each food group every day to ensure that your child is getting a balance of all the nutrients required to grow and develop. Keep introducing new foods. Once they have passed their first birthday children may be a little more reluctant to try them.

Fat

Fat provides the most concentrated source of energy. Infants need more fat in their diets than adults to support their rapid growth and development. Your baby will be unable to eat a large enough volume of low-fat food to meet energy requirements. Full-fat dairy food products, such as cheese and yogurt, are recommended at this stage. Use full-fat vegetable margarine or butter on bread and vegetables and add to potato or pasta.

Sugar

Giving your child foods high in sugar will encourage a sweet tooth. This doesn't mean that such foods should never be given. They are less damaging to teeth if they are taken at the end of meals.

Snacks

Since it is difficult for a child to achieve enough energy and nutrients in just 3 meals a day snacks or milk should be offered twice a day between meals. If snacks are well spaced between meals they will not affect your child's appetite.

sample menu for 1-year-old child (end stage 4)

Mid-morning/mid-afternoon/evening (2–3 times a day)

☐ Breast feed or a drink of formula from a cup.

☐ Other drink cooled boiled tap water from a cup with each meal.

Breakfast

Any of the following

☐ breakfast cereal e.g. Weetabix, Ready Brek or porridge with full-fat cow's milk and finely chopped fruit

☐ wholemeal bread/toast and yogurt with finely chopped fruit

☐ scrambled egg on wholemeal toast and chopped tomato.

Lunch (or light meal)

☐ Bread, toast, pitta bread, pasta or crackers with meat, cheese, eggs, tuna, tinned salmon or hummus, and fruit and salad vegetables

Dessert

☐ fruit yogurt or fromage frais

Dinner (or main meal)

Any of the following

☐ chicken or lamb casserole with sweet potato and selection of vegetables

☐ spaghetti bolognese topped with grated cheese

☐ risotto with mushroom, mangetout and fish or meat pieces

☐ baked potato with beans and cheese

☐ mashed potato and pork chops cut in pieces with turnip

Dessert

Any of the following

☐ soft fresh fruit quarters, e.g. banana, pear, melon (no seeds)

☐ stewed fruit, e.g. apples, apricots (with stones removed)

☐ tinned soft fruit in natural juice, e.g. pear, peaches

☐ semolina with chopped soft fruits

☐ yogurt or fromage frais (full-fat varieties)

Snacks (for between meals)

☐ plain scones halved, bread or toast soldiers, unsalted crackers, pancakes, croissant

☐ chopped fruit and vegetables, e.g. chunks of peach, banana or peeled and cored whole apple or pear, thin slices of melon, sticks of carrot or cucumber

☐ natural yogurt or plain fromage frais — add your own fruit

☐ cheese, milk (maximum 600 mls a day in total)

Occasional snacks (containing a lot of sugar)

☐ flavoured yogurt, flavoured fromage frais

☐ plain biscuits, e.g. digestive, rich tea

Mealtime routines

Establish a routine for your child with 3 main meal times of breakfast, lunch and dinner each day. This will make your child feel happy and secure and he or she will eat more.

Eat together as a family as much as possible, or at least have those present together at meal times. Your child will watch everything and learn a lot. Mealtimes should be fun—relaxed and not strained—otherwise children may associate mealtimes with something they do not enjoy.

Drinks

Continue to give breastfeeds between meals or approximately 500–600 mls (17–20 oz) of infant formula milk a day, encouraging your child to drink it from a cup as much as possible. After your child's first birthday cow's milk can be used as the main milk drink, but limit it to 600 mls (approximately 1 pint) a day. Offer a small volume of cooled boiled tap water from a cup with meals.

Drinks

Breast milk, formula and cooled boiled water

Breast milk or infant formula and water are the only drinks that should be given to babies under 12 months and should continue to be the main drinks given during the first year of life. Breastfeeding or formula milk feeds need to continue during weaning.

Water

If additional fluid is needed apart from breast or formula milk, water (cooled, pre-boiled, up to the age of 6 months, thereafter freshly drawn) is the best option. Water and milk are the only two drinks necessary. They won't damage teeth or provoke a desire for sweet foods.

Cow's milk

Cow's milk should not be given to your child as a drink before the age of 12 months. Full-fat (whole) cow's milk can, however, be mixed into foods such as custard, rice pudding and mashed potato, and cereal, preferably from 6 months onwards (although it can be added to solids from 4 months). Full-fat milk can be used as a main drink from 1 year of age. Low-fat (semi-skimmed) cow's milk is suitable from 2 years of age provided your child is thriving and eating a good varied diet. Skimmed milk is not appropriate for any child under the age of 5 and possibly older.

Don't add sugar, honey, rusks, baby rice or other cereals and food to your baby's bottle or cup of milk. It may interfere with the amount of milk your baby drinks and deprive him or her of the opportunity to learn to take food from a spoon as well as harming teeth.

Fruit juices

Fruit juices are not necessary for babies but if you do give them, remember the following points.

- Offer juice from a cup not a bottle.
- Don't replace infant formula with juice.
- Use sparingly; give a small volume of juice from a cup at one meal.
- Be careful not to let your baby drink more than needed; the tummy will fill up resulting in a poor appetite for more nutritious solid food.
- Pure fruit juices are not normally suitable before 6 months and thereafter need to be well diluted with fresh water (1 part juice mixed with 5–10 parts freshly drawn tap water).
- Baby juices and baby herbal drinks contain sugar (up to 9 g per 100 mls, which is similar to the amount of sugar in a soft drink). They can damage developing teeth. If given too often the baby may reject water as a drink and develop a preference for sweet foods.
- Avoid fruit squashes as they often contain artificial additives such as sweeteners and colourings, which are not permitted in baby foods.

Unsuitable drinks for infants

- Drinks with artificial sweeteners, e.g. aspartame and saccharin, for children under 3 years of age.
- Tea and coffee: they contain tannin which binds with iron and other minerals and reduces their absorption by the body.
- Carbonated or fizzy drinks are acidic and can erode tooth enamel and lead to tooth decay. Due to their unpredictable composition, they are unsuitable for infants.
- Cola and several other carbonated drinks contain stimulants such as caffeine.
- Soft drinks have a high sugar content; most range between 8 and 11 g per 100 mls.
- Natural mineral water and spring water, whether still or carbonated, may contain high levels of sodium and minerals, which make them unsuitable for infants and toddlers. The majority are also unsuitable for making up formula. Fizzy or carbonated bottled water is acidic and so may damage teeth.

If you have to use bottled water for making up your baby's bottles e.g. if tap water is unsuitable or unsafe to drink when on holidays or otherwise, use still mineral water and check the nutritional label to ensure that the sodium (Na+) content is less than 200 mg per 1000 mls (1 litre).

Boil the water before use. See Chapter 5, pages 57–8, for feed preparation guidelines, but never re-boil water for formula preparation.

Don't let your baby fall asleep or leave him or her alone with a bottle or beaker in the mouth.

If there is a family history of allergy

> ### positive family history of allergy
>
> When one or more of a baby's first-degree relatives i.e. parent or sibling, suffer from asthma, eczema, hay fever or food allergy, the baby has a positive family history of allergy.

If there is a confirmed or positive family history of allergies it is best to breastfeed your baby. Exclusive breastfeeding for 4 to 6 months is the most effective dietary measure for the prevention of allergies.

Don't start weaning until your baby is at least 4 months old. Start with the least allergenic foods i.e. baby rice, root vegetables, fruit (see first foods, pages 67–8).

Once your baby is taking these foods, potentially allergenic foods i.e. cow's milk, egg, soya, peanuts, tree nuts, wheat and fish can be introduced. There is no evidence that there is any benefit to delaying or excluding these foods, and indeed new research suggests that avoiding allergenic foods may actually increase the risk of developing an allergy to them. It is recommended however, that you introduce high-allergenic foods one by one, leaving a gap of 3 days in between each one. See Chapter 13 for further details.

If weaning is delayed or foods are excluded from your baby's diet you should ask a dietitian to assess the nutritional adequacy of the diet.

Weaning on to a vegetarian or vegan diet

Vegetarian

Weaning on to a vegetarian diet requires extra planning to ensure your baby achieves enough energy, protein, vitamins, iron and other minerals, all of which are essential for a small baby.

You should either breastfeed or give a suitable infant formula until your child is 2 years old. If your baby is bottle-fed, it is better to change to a follow-on formula from 6 months of age e.g. Aptamil Follow-on, SMA Follow-on, or Cow & Gate Follow-on Milk.

To begin with, follow the guidelines for stage 1 of weaning, pages 67–8. Vegetarian babies can start with the usual combination of fruits, vegetables and cereals. After about 2 weeks of weaning, at stage 2, you will need to offer alternatives for meat and chicken such as puréed pulses.

Then, as variety and texture increase at stage 3 the following foods should be included:

- Well-cooked eggs; the white and yolk should be solid
- Cheese
- Tahini-sesame seed paste
- Smooth nut-paste (always spread nut paste thinly on e.g. bread, never offer from a teaspoon as chunks of smooth nut paste, particularly if the paste is dry, can pose a choking hazard; avoid whole or chopped nuts until the age of 5)
- Soya protein (TVP)
- Mashed or minced quorn
- Hummus
- Tofu

Tip Add extra cereal, breast or formula milk, margarine or oil to weaning food to increase its energy density.

Poor weight gain is a risk for vegetarian infants. Vegetarian diets can be relatively high in fibre which can fill a baby's stomach before enough calories are consumed. Fibre can reduce the absorption of some important minerals, such as iron and zinc. Iron from non-meat sources is less well absorbed. See Chapter 14 for further information.

Vegan

Vegan diets present an even bigger and more complex challenge than vegetarian diets in terms of providing sufficient nutrition for babies and children. Such diets are not recommended by medical experts. It is not easy for your baby to obtain the nutrition vital for adequate growth, health and development on a vegan diet. See Chapter 14 for further information.

Useful equipment

There is such a dazzling array of feeding-related items available in the shops you may feel you need to spend a large sum of money, but simple utensils are all that are needed. The following are the essentials, some of which you may already have in your kitchen.

Baby spoons Buy some shallow plastic weaning spoons for feeding your baby; they are flatter and smaller than regular spoons. Many have long handles to reach easily into jars, some are heat sensitive and change colour when food is too hot.

At around 6 months of age babies want to try holding their own spoon, so have an extra one handy at mealtimes. However, it will be a few more months before co-ordination has developed enough for your baby to get food from the bowl to the mouth with a spoon.

Plates and bowls Small durable plastic bowls in bright colours, that are dishwasher safe are good for serving meals. Or you can simply use the lid of a baby bottle initially. Babies sometimes throw their bowls and dinner on the floor; bowls with suction cups on the bottom are available if you wish.

Liquidiser or blender A liquidiser or food processor is useful for puréeing large quantities of food. A hand blender may be useful for smaller quantities. Purées can be prepared very quickly and easily with any of these. However, purées for young babies will often need to be sieved afterwards to remove any seeds, pips or skins.

Fork and sieve A simple fork and a metal sieve can be used to purée a small portion of food. Use a fork to mash the food, then press it through the sieve to get rid of the lumps, seeds or skins. The texture can then be adjusted as necessary with some liquid.

Ice-cube tray, freezer bags and small plastic containers with lids Ice-cube trays are great for the first few weeks while you are introducing your baby to new tastes. Food placed into a flexible plastic ice cube trays can be frozen, then the cubes can be pushed out and put into freezer bags. Simply defrost one or two cubes as required. As your baby begins to eat more, plastic containers with lids or even yogurt cartons covered with cling film are useful.

Cups Trainer cups should be introduced when your baby is 6 months old. Choose one with two handles then let your baby hold it by him or herself as soon as he or she is able, or wants to do so—it will be good practice. Lidded beakers are very popular and especially handy when out and about. However, an open cup will encourage a more mature suck or tongue motion although your baby may need a little more help initially. Aim for your child to have finished drinking from a bottle around the first birthday.

High chair Your baby will need somewhere safe and comfortable (not to mention washable) to sit during mealtimes. Babies need to be in a good position to manage spoon feeds. At around 4 months old, your baby will be able to sit in a high chair so you should invest in or borrow a wooden, metal or plastic high chair. A high chair with a tray is good for feeding as it encourages your baby to sit upright and play with the food before trying or eating it.

Ensure your baby can bring his or her hands together to touch the food on the tray. To prevent your baby slumping wrap a towel, or some other soft washable object around his or her middle.

Place the high chair at the dinner table when others are eating; your baby will enjoy the social interaction and will also adapt to the mealtime routine and learn a lot by looking around at everyone eating.

A booster seat, which straps to your own dining chairs, is more portable than a high chair and takes up less space but may not be as stable or as comfortable as a high chair. Booster seats are more suited to older babies and toddlers.

Homemade weaning food

If you prepare your own weaning food you know exactly what goes into it. Your baby will become used to the taste of adult type foods and will accept a broader range of tastes and textures as a toddler and young child. It is as if that early exposure helps to programme the palate.

Homemade weaning foods are cheap to prepare and there is very little waste if you prepare and freeze a batch of meals. Although it takes much longer to prepare meals than to buy them it is only at the early stages of weaning that you need to prepare your baby's meals separately from your own meals.

Meat, poultry, fish (make sure to remove all bones) or pulses can be stewed, baked, steamed or boiled as for the rest of the family. Cook thoroughly until tender before puréeing.

It is so important to introduce these protein sources early i.e. 2–4 weeks after weaning starts. Combine them with puréed vegetables, rice or potato, adjusting the texture with the usual milk. Avoid mixing with gravy and packet or jarred sauce, as they contain a lot of salt. Baby rice is a good thickener for purées that are too thin.

Freezing baby food

Your time is precious so don't waste it by preparing individual puréed meals. Cook more than needed once or twice a week and freeze the extra servings in ice-cubes trays or small plastic containers. Cook the food then purée, cover and cool quickly.

Most foods freeze well except banana, melon and baby rice.

For young babies freeze in small quantities. Pour the cooled purée into a flexible sterile ice cube tray, wrap in a freezer bag and leave in the freezer for 4 hours. Then take the tray from the freezer and knock out the food cubes into a labelled and dated freezer bag and return to freezer. Remember to label the meals and write the date by which they should be used. Baby foods can be stored in a freezer for up to 8 weeks. Small plastic cartons or containers can be used as the amount eaten increases.

Seal both plastic freezer bags and cartons well, extract as much air as possible or fill cartons to the top as this will help prevent the food drying out.

Refreezing baby food, for example after prolonged power cuts, is not safe. It's always best to discard it.

cooking fruit and vegetables

Fruit

- Always examine fruit before preparing it for cooking. The riper it is the less water and heat needed to soften or cook it. If the fruit is extremely ripe it may not need to be cooked.
- Wash the fruit under running cold water then peel, seed or stone it. Cut into 6 or 8 triangles through the core (discard the core and pips).
- Steaming fruit may result in some of the actual fruit and juice running through the holes of the steamer and being lost so it is better to stew it. Use a small amount of water, about 2 cm (just over ½ inch) in the saucepan. When the fruit is soft purée it. Correct the consistency as necessary with a little breast milk or formula milk.
- When using a microwave use as little water as possible or no water at all especially if the fruit is soft. Cover the food with cling film, leaving a small air vent and cook on full power (stop and stir half way through). Purée to the desired consistency. Check that it is not too hot before serving and stir well to avoid hot spots.

Vegetables

- Wash vegetables under cold running water. Peel, trim and slice. Steaming vegetables until tender minimises the loss of vitamins and minerals. When the vegetable is soft purée or mash as appropriate. Correct the consistency as necessary with a little breast milk or formula milk
- When boiling vegetables use as little water as possible—barely cover the vegetables. Be careful not to overcook. Some of the cooking liquid can be used to make the vegetable into a smooth purée.
- To achieve a totally smooth texture after liquidising or puréeing, some fruit or vegetables may need to be passed/forked through a metal sieve to remove any residual pips or seeds.

Defrosting

Leave frozen food covered in the fridge overnight to defrost. Thaw foods as needed for the following day—one or more cubes or a carton. If you forget to leave food out of the freezer the night before, leave it out at room temperature, make sure it is covered and transfer it into the fridge once defrosted. Don't place food in warm water to defrost. Always use defrosted foods within 24 hours.

how to make gravy suitable for babies

Mix 120 mls vegetable water (with no added salt) with 2 small teaspoons corn flour and half a teaspoon tomato purée. Heat until the mixture thickens, stir and allow to cool.

Reheating

Don't reheat food more than once. Make sure the food is completely thawed then heat in a small saucepan or microwave right the way through, stirring well, especially if microwaving. Reheated food must be piping hot the whole way through to kill the bacteria in it. Then leave it to cool to prevent burning your baby's mouth. Always check the temperature before serving or feeding food to your baby.

Fruit and vegetable purées and baby rice

Vegetable purées A range of vegetables can be used to make your own purées—parsnip, turnip, butternut squash, broccoli, cauliflower, courgette, peas, leek. Each of these vegetables can be prepared in the same way as carrot (below). Some vegetables will also require sieving to remove any skin, pips etc., e.g. peas. Serve individually or try mixing two together for variety or try combining a vegetable with a fruit e.g. parsnip and apple. If the vegetable purée is too thin stir in some baby rice to thicken it.

Fruit purées Always use ripe fruit when making purées. Remove any small pips and stones. Some purées e.g. banana, melon, don't need to be cooked. Many fruits are slightly acid or tart e.g. rhubarb. Don't add sugar to sweeten but instead serve them with a bland food e.g. baby rice or rice purée (see recipe on following page) which will give a creamier finish.

Baby rice Ground (baby) rice has a fine texture, is easily digested and is gluten free. Its milky taste makes for an easy transition to solids.

Carrot purée

2 medium carrots (provides 4 portions.)

Wash the vegetable under a running cold tap. Peel, trim and slice. Steam until tender (15–25 minutes), boil in approximately 3 cm of water or add a little water, cover with cling film and microwave until soft. Purée in a blender. Blend with your baby's usual milk to give the correct consistency or use the cooking liquid if boiled.

Pear purée

2 small ripe pears (provides 5 portions)

Wash the fruit under a running cold tap. Peel, quarter and core. Stew in a little water until soft (about 5 minutes). Purée in a blender. Adjust the texture with milk to make it runnier or baby rice to make it stiffer.

Banana purée

½ ripe banana (provides 1 portion)

Peel and purée in a blender, adding milk to soften.

mix flavours

Early meals can be made more interesting by mixing different purées together or with one or two other ingredients: e.g. mix baby rice with puréed apple, banana, carrot, or broccoli or mix a fruit with a vegetable purée e.g. parsnip and apple or mix two vegetable purées e.g. carrot and pea or 2–3 fruit purées e.g. apricot and pear, pear, apple and banana.

home-made foods have more flavour

Commercial foods are perfectly acceptable and are useful when travelling or eating away from home but try to use home-prepared foods as much as possible. Home-made foods expose babies to more flavours and a wider variety of family foods and as result babies tend to be less fussy about food as they grow up.

organic baby food
Approximately half of all commercial baby food sold is organic and is free from artificial additives, hydrogenated fats and genetically modified ingredients.

Commercial baby rice

Mix the baby rice with cooled boiled water, breast or infant formula milk.

Home-made rice purée

1 tablespoon ground rice (provides 1 portion)

250 mls baby's usual milk

Mix the ground rice with the milk, a little at a time. Pour into a saucepan and bring to the boil, stirring. Simmer until cooked (5–8 minutes), stirring occasionally.

food hygiene

Babies and young children are more vulnerable to severe illness from food-borne infection than older children or adults. So you need to take great care to ensure that all foods are fresh, clean, hygienically prepared and stored correctly.

- Always wash your hands before and during food preparation.
- Ensure ingredients are fresh or within the manufacturer's best before date.
- Sterilise plastic serving bowls, spoons, sieve, ice-cube trays or freezer containers and the removable parts of the blender until your baby is 6 months old to avoid infection. This can done by boiling utensils in a saucepan of water for 5 minutes or soaking them in a pan with Milton or another baby safe sterilising solution, following the manufacturer's instructions.
- If you have a steam steriliser, small items such as spoons or serving bowls can be sterilised following the manufacturer's guidelines.
- Use a dishwasher if you have one, as the temperature reached is much higher than can be tolerated when hand washing.
- Dry everything with kitchen paper or leave to drip dry.
- Meals prepared in advance can be kept covered and in the fridge for a maximum of 24 hours before discarding.
- Partly eaten food must be discarded as it will have been contaminated with saliva and bacteria will grow.
- Both parent and baby should start meals with clean hands.

EU guidelines
All commercial baby foods have to comply with strict EU guidelines on nutritional content. Each product is labelled with instructions for use, the ingredients and the nutritional information.

Shop-bought baby foods

Shop-bought or commercial baby foods are widely available and offer a convenient alternative to home-cooked meals, especially when travelling and eating away from home. Most parents use these foods at some stage during weaning because they are so convenient. They are also relatively expensive.

These foods have to conform to strict regulations regarding safety, composition and added vitamins and minerals. They are sterile before opening. However, always check that the seal is intact and that the product is within its best before date.

Nutritional content

It is worth checking the protein content of shop-bought foods. You will find it in the nutritional information section on each of the jars or boxes. Look for the figure per 100 g, not per jar. With dried baby food, look for the amount per 100 g of 'made up' food, not per 100 g of dried food.

Meat or fish dishes should contain at least 2.5 g protein per 100 g. Vegetable savouries should contain at least 2 g protein per 100 g. Sweet meals should contain at least 1 g protein per 100 g.

Other information is given, such as that the food is totally meat free and suitable for vegetarians or it is gluten free. There is often a tick-list at the side of baby jars indicating if the food is gluten free, milk free, has no added sugar etc.

It is best to choose savoury meals rather than sweetened desserts and puddings. The sugar content of desserts can be quite high, e.g. from almost 9 g of sugar for a serving of traditional egg custard, to over 15 g for some of the other dessert pots.

baby jars, both savoury and sweet, containing smooth purées are usually labelled 'suitable from 4 months old' (stage 1); jars with purées containing small lumps, are usually labelled 'suitable from 7 months old' (stage 3).

dried foods, both savoury and sweet, require reconstitution with a suitable liquid such as cooled boiled water or breast or formula milk.

cereal based foods are available in jars e.g. baby porridge or as dried product e.g. baby rice, semolina.

Don't rely too much on commercial baby foods

Although in the early stages of weaning many parents opt for the convenience of dried manufactured foods try to introduce the taste of real vegetables and fruit to your baby as early as possible so that he or she acquires a taste for these foods and goes on eating them when older. There is a proven link between early food experience (exposure) and subsequent food acceptance.

Try not to use commercial foods every day as they taste blander than home-made food and this may discourage your baby from expanding his or her taste range. In addition, keeping your infant on puréed baby foods for prolonged periods may delay acceptance of more lumpy foods.

7 Common infant feeding problems

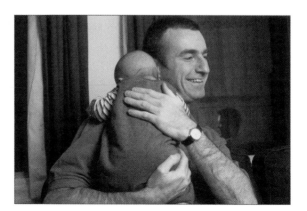

During a baby's first year some problems with feeding may arise. Most of these are minor and can be managed at home but they can be distressing for both babies and parents. If you are concerned, it is better to visit the doctor or public health nurse than to sit at home worrying. Early intervention and treatment are central to your baby's health and wellbeing.

Sometimes a GP may have little experience dealing with babies. If you are not happy with the outcome of your visit it may be worth looking for a second opinion. Remember, nobody knows your baby as well as you do.

In this chapter we advise on how to cope with common feeding problems that are not too serious.

Wind

Wind affects all babies to some extent as they usually swallow air while feeding. When feeds are taken too slowly or too quickly, the amount of air swallowed may increase. Babies may also swallow air while crying and even while breathing. While this is perfectly normal, too much trapped wind in the tummy can make babies feel uncomfortable and full. A baby suffering from wind may stop feeding and cry, or squirm or have a pained expression on the face.

Babies vary in how often they need to be winded during feeding. Some babies have very little wind and may only need to be winded at the end of a feed, or not at all, while others need to be winded quite regularly e.g. after every 2 oz of feed or at any stage during the feed when they become uncomfortable.

Babies also differ in how easily they bring up their wind. Some babies will bring it up within a minute or two in a nice satisfying burp but others take longer.

How to wind a baby

At the end of a feed, or during a feed if you see signs of discomfort, place your baby over your shoulder, or sitting on your lap, or face down on your lap. Then hold the baby firmly with one hand and use the other hand to pat or rub his or her back gently but firmly until the wind comes up in one or a number of burps.

One position may suit your baby more than the others. In each case it is important to keep the baby's back nice and straight.

Positions for winding

- Against your body, with the baby's head over your shoulder: place the baby against your shoulder with his or her bottom supported by your arm on that side. Pat or rub the back gently but firmly with the other hand.
- Sitting up: sit the baby on your lap facing to the side and leaning forward; gently cup his or her chin in your hand. Pat or rub the baby's back gently but firmly with the other hand.
- Face-down on your lap: place the baby face down on your lap and hold firmly with one hand. Pat or rub the baby's back gently but firmly with the other hand.

Don't spend longer than a few minutes at the end of a feed trying to get your baby's wind up. Your baby may well settle to sleep without bringing up any wind. Sometimes a baby will pass flatus rather than burping.

Wind in breastfed babies

In general, breastfed babies have fewer problems with wind than those on bottle feeds. This is because they can control the flow of milk at the breast. However, in the first few weeks of life breastfed babies may not be able to make a good lip seal around the nipple and they swallow air during sucking. Also, if a breast-fed baby is a fast feeder, or if the milk flow from the breast is particularly quick, wind may be a problem.

Tips for reducing wind in a breastfed baby

- Ensure the baby has a good seal around the nipple, i.e. is properly attached (see Chapter 3, pages 29–30).
- Consider having your GP, midwife or public health nurse check your baby for tongue tie. Babies who are tongue tied can find it difficult to latch on. This can result in feeding difficulties for the baby and significant discomfort for the mother.
- Use a nipple shield (available from pharmacies) to slow down the flow of milk if the flow is too fast and the baby is gulping in both milk and air.
- Observe the effect on your baby of the different foods you eat. For example, spicy food upsets some babies while it is perfectly tolerated by others. It is a matter of trial and error.

Tips for reducing wind in a bottle-fed baby

- Ensure the flow rate from the teat suits the baby—see Chapter 5, page 53.
- Tilt the bottle so the teat and bottle neck are constantly full of milk.
- Allow the bottle to stand until all the air bubbles produced by shaking have settled before giving the feed to your baby. If this takes too long, instead of shaking the bottle, swirl it for several seconds.
- Position the baby a little more upright during feeding.
- Don't let the baby suck on the bottle when the feed is finished or when only milk bubbles are left.
- Give smaller, more frequent feeds.

Colic

Colic affects up to 30 per cent of babies, usually at between 3 and 13 weeks of age. It affects breastfed and formula-fed babies equally. A baby with colic has spells of unexplained irritability, agitation, fussing or crying. The main symptom is non-stop inconsolable crying, without any obvious cause. Not surprisingly, colic causes a great deal of stress in families.

Babies with colic often cry at around the same time of day, usually after their afternoon or evening feeds. They may bring their knees up to their chest as if in pain, become tense, go red in the face and may also be windy.

Crying is one of the ways a baby communicates that they are tired, hungry, over-stimulated or simply want to release tension. However, a baby with infant colic cannot be comforted during crying episodes. Sometimes a baby with colic will writhe in pain and cry inconsolably and it is important to check that there is no medical cause for this by bringing your baby to the GP. A diagnosis of colic is usually made when no other problem can be found and the baby is otherwise well and growing normally. If you suspect your baby has colic it is a good idea to take him or her to the GP for a physical examination.

possible common causes of colic
- Build up of wind
- Over-stimulation

less common causes
- Lactose intolerance
- Cow's milk protein allergy

Try keeping a diary of crying episodes to check for a pattern. It is also worth remembering that most people experience abdominal pain before examinations or interviews—there is little doubt that stress felt by parents or caregivers is transmitted to babies.

Causes of colic

Medical research has failed to find the exact cause of colic, but a combination of factors is likely to be responsible. It is widely thought that painful contractions of the gut due to a build-up of wind may be a cause and that the baby's crying, drawing up of legs and so on are probably due to pain. Wind may accumulate if your baby swallows air when feeding or crying. Painful gut contractions may also be caused by cow's milk protein intolerance or lactose intolerance. Over-stimulation is another possible cause.

if you can't console your crying baby
Try rhythmic stimulation by placing the baby near a vibrating appliance such as a tumble drier or washing machine (when not on the spin cycle!), or in a bouncy chair or make a short car journey or push the baby repeatedly forwards and backwards in the pram.

Treatment of colic

There is no single correct way to deal with colic. The only proven treatment is time. Most colicky babies outgrow the problem between 4 and 6 months of age but this is of little consolation to parents of a young baby when a half hour of inconsolable crying can seem like an eternity. It's worth trying the following:

- Check the baby is not hungry or thirsty.
- If you are bottle-feeding try making up bottles with 1–2 oz more than you think the baby will drink. This will allow feeding to appetite and you will know that the baby is full when he or she stops feeding.
- If you are breastfeeding don't switch to the second breast too quickly while the first still has milk to give. Hind milk contains more fat than fore milk. Fat slows down stomach emptying and lactose is released more slowly into the small bowel thus aiding digestion.
- Carry and gently rock the baby. Sometimes babies get bored or simply want some extra attention and a cuddle.
- Try to reduce the baby's wind as discussed above.
- Offer feeds more often.
- Offer the baby a soother. There are times when a baby is not hungry but wants to suck on something for comfort and soothers can be useful. (If you are breastfeeding it is best not to offer a soother until breastfeeding has been established.)
- Place a warm face cloth or hot water bottle wrapped in a towel on the baby's tummy (make sure the hot water bottle does not feel too hot).
- Relax the baby by giving a warm bath.
- Try gently massaging your baby's tummy in a circular clockwise motion about an hour before you think he or she is likely to start crying—but not just after a feed. Use a baby massage oil.

Note It is best to work through these suggestions in a sequence over a few hours or days, deciding yourself which one to try first. Bear in mind none of them may work.

Steps to reduce over-stimulation

Babies can be over-stimulated by too much loud noise, bright lights or the presence of several people at one time. Some babies are prone to over-stimulation due to an immature central nervous system. The following measures to reduce over-stimulation may be helpful in the management of colic:

- Minimise loud household noises.
- Place the baby in a dark quiet room.
- Swaddle the baby by wrapping snugly in a blanket or sheet. This technique is often used in hospitals and may also be helpful if the baby is over tired or needs to feel snug. If you're unsure how to do it ask your public health nurse or an experienced friend. Most babies like to be swaddled up until 6 weeks of age and sometimes longer. If the baby becomes agitated and fights being so tightly wrapped you will know that the time has come to stop. It is also important to make sure that the baby is not too warm.

Lactase deficiency

Your baby may develop a temporary mild lactase deficiency so that the lactose in the formula or breast milk will not be properly digested and may cause colicky pain. It is not possible to test for lactase deficiency as a cause of colic but if your baby has colic it is worth trying a low-lactose formula or giving lactase drops. (See Chapter 8, page 111.)

If a low-lactose feed fails to reduce colic then the final option for treatment is a 1–2 week trial on a hypoallergenic formula such as Nutramigen (by Mead Johnson) or Aptamil Pepti.

Cow's milk protein allergy

In a small number of cases colic may be caused by a cow's milk protein allergy. This is more likely if there is a family history of allergy. Try a hypoallergenic formula such as Nutramigen or Aptamil Pepti for 1–2 weeks. If the baby responds to the formula discuss with your doctor, public health nurse or dietitian how long to continue with it. Breastfeeding mothers should consider a two-week trial on a dairy-free diet. It is essential that all sources of dairy are removed from the diet. Milk is added to many different products and hidden sources of milk include some brands of sausages and beef burgers, some crisps and some breakfast cereals. However, removing foods from the diet significantly increases the risk of nutritional deficiencies so should only be done under medical supervision. Ideally, you should obtain advice from a dietitian especially if you are going to continue on a milk-free diet for a number of weeks or you have to avoid more than one food type.

gripe water, Dentinox and Infacol have not been scientifically proven to help in cases of infant colic. However, some parents have found them beneficial and there is no evidence that they cause any harm.

Dairy products are a very valuable source of calcium, protein and vitamin B_{12} and you will need to find alternative sources of these nutrients if you go on a dairy-free diet.

Other treatments for colic

A number of treatments for colic are available from pharmacies, including Infacol, Dentinox and gripe water. However, none has been scientifically proven to be effective.

Infacol contains the active ingredient simeticone. Simeticone is a deflatulent which helps bring up wind or air trapped in the tummy. It makes small gas bubbles join into bigger bubbles which are easier to burp. It is given before each feed and is suitable from birth onwards.

Dentinox Infant Colic Drops work in a similar way to Infacol. Unlike Infacol the drops can be added to the baby's bottle or they can be taken from a spoon either with or after a feed. It should not be given more than 6 times a day. It is suitable from birth onwards.

Gripe water Alcohol-free gripe water is no longer available in the Republic of Ireland (in essence because the market is too small) but continues to be sold in the UK including Northern Ireland. It can also be bought online from the UK website www.auravita.com. (Delivery charges can be reduced by using a virtual UK address service provided by companies such as Parcel Motel, DPD or An Post.) Gripe water contains sodium hydrogen carbonate, which helps neutralise stomach acids, and dill seed oil, which helps dissipate trapped air. It is sugar and alcohol free. It is not suitable for infants under 4 weeks. Gripe water is given from a spoon either during or after each feed.

Herbal remedies

Some mothers have reported herbal remedies such as fennel, chamomile and balm mint drinks to be helpful. These herbs have been shown to have an anti-spasmodic activity. However, not all herbal remedies are safe and they should be used with caution.

Many people mistakenly believe that because herbal remedies are 'natural' they must automatically be safe. Some herbal remedies work in the same way as licensed drugs but do not have to undergo any rigorous safety checks before they are sold to the public. It is best to speak with your doctor or public health nurse before trying a new product. It is also important to ensure that any herbal drinks given to babies are sugar free.

rest and relaxation
It is important for parents to take a break from time to time. Where possible ask friends or family to take care of your baby for brief periods to give you some time to refresh and recharge your batteries. Look for help if you have trouble coping. It can be very hard caring for a baby who cries for long spells every day.

make your own herbal drink
Add some fennel and mint leaves to water, bring to the boil for a few minutes and strain. Offer this drink to the baby once it has cooled to lukewarm. It is best to make it up fresh each time and give no more than 30 mls (1 oz) twice a day.

Constipation

Constipation is one of the most common problems seen in paediatric out-patient departments but reassuringly, it is usually only a temporary problem, not associated with any underlying disease.

Constipation is very rare in breastfed infants as breast milk tends to have a mild laxative effect. It is more common in bottle-fed infants. Remember that babies' bowel habits vary considerably and it is easy to have an unrealistic idea of what's normal. It is important to be able to recognise a normal bowel habit as it is not uncommon for people to have very different ideas about what is normal!

Normal stool

Breastfed babies Stools are runny or soft and seedy. They can vary in colour from yellow or mustard to orange with little white flecks that look like seeds. It can be normal for a breastfed baby to stool after every feed or, once breastfeeding is established and the baby is older than 6 weeks, as infrequently as once a week.

Bottle-fed babies Stools are usually a soft paste (more formed than a breastfed babies) though sometimes they can be runny. They can vary in colour, depending on the type of formula, from greyish-green to yellow, tan or brown. It can be normal for bottle-fed babies to stool from once to three times a day to once every two to three days.

Babies taking solids It is normal for the stools of breast- and bottle-fed babies to change once they start on solids. The stools can vary from a paste to a formed consistency and often contain undigested food. The colour varies depending on what is eaten. Bowel motions may be less frequent once solids have been started, especially for breast-fed babies.

Note Once older than 6 weeks, it can be normal for exclusively breastfed babies to go for 7–10 days without a bowel motion; 2–3 days without a motion can be normal for some bottle-fed babies.

causes of constipation in infants
- Dietary change
- Inadequate fluid intake
- Incorrect feed preparation
- Cow's milk protein allergy (there are no tests for this)
- Unknown

Constipated stools

The stools are firm, dry and pellet like. They do not soak into the nappy but are dry lumps.

While constipation can often result in less frequent bowel motions compared to normal, it is the consistency or the hardness of the stool that is the most important factor in determining whether a baby is constipated or not.

Straining

Straining at stool can be normal for babies but straining with crying can be a sign of constipation.

Causes of constipation in infants

1. Dietary change

Babies' guts are very sensitive and any dietary change such as switching formula or introducing a new food may result in changes in the consistency and frequency of the stool. It may take a few days for the baby's gut to adjust to a new food or formula. If after a few days the baby's bowel motions remain unsatisfactory, it is probably better to change back to the old formula or offer a combination of the old and new formulas.

It is perfectly safe to mix two different formulas together. Prepare the formulas in the usual way and then mix them together, for example, prepare 120 ml (4 oz) of each formula and mix together to give a 240 ml (8 oz) bottle. Sometimes you may need to mix a bigger volume of the old formula with a smaller volume of the new formula, for example, 180 ml (6 oz) of the old and 60 ml (2 oz) of the new formula. The volume of new formula can then be slowly increased over a few days or a week.

If constipation develops at 1 year of age following the introduction of cow's milk it may be a good idea to switch back to infant formula for a few weeks or alternatively you could mix cow's milk and infant formula together.

If a new food is the suspected culprit avoid giving it for a few weeks. There is anecdotal evidence to suggest that baby rice and bananas can be constipating. There is no scientific rationale for this and most babies who eat these foods will not experience any problems.

If a breastfed baby develops constipation on the introduction of formula milk it may be useful to offer a combination of breast and formula feeds for a time. First milks may be easier on the baby's digestive system than second or follow on milks. Alternatively the formulas Cow & Gate Comfort, SMA Comfort or Aptamil Comfort may be of benefit.

2. Inadequate fluid intake

Inadequate fluid intake is the most common cause of constipation in infants. During the first 6 months of life breast milk or infant formula is the only fluid a baby needs. Babies under 6 months need approximately 150 mls per kg per day; babies of 6 months and over need 120 mls per kg per day. The ready reckoner below will help you to check if your baby is getting enough fluid. Sometimes even an extra 1–2 oz fluid a day helps improve constipation.

If you are concerned about your baby's intake of formula or breast milk speak to your doctor, public health nurse, practice nurse or dietitian.

Fluid ready reckoner	
Baby's weight	Average volume of feed that needs to be taken over 24 hours
3.0 kg or 6 lbs 9½ oz	450 mls or 15 oz
4.0 kg or 8 lbs 13 oz	600 mls or 20 oz
5.0 kg or 11 lbs	750 mls or 25 oz
6.0 kg or 13 lbs 3 oz	900 mls or 30 oz
7.0 kg or 15 lbs or 6½ oz	840 mls or 28 oz
8.0 kg or 17lbs 9½ oz	960 mls or 32 oz
9.0 kg or 19 lbs 13 oz	1080 mls 36 oz

3. Incorrect feed preparation

If a feed is slightly over concentrated this can be a cause of constipation. When preparing infant formula the boiled water should always be added to the bottle first. One level scoop of formula powder for every 1 fl oz or 30 mls of water gives the correct feed concentration. It is important not to use more or less than this unless it has been recommended by a dietitian. Scoops should not be swapped from one type or brand of formula to another as they may not be the same size. It is also important not to compress the powder when levelling off a scoop.

4. Cow's milk protein allergy

This is a rare cause of constipation and should only be considered in babies who develop chronic or persistent constipation following the introduction of cow's milk-based formula and where the constipation fails to respond to conventional treatment.

There are no tests for cow's milk protein allergy as a potential cause of constipation. The only way to check is to remove all sources of cow's milk from the diet and observe the baby for signs of improvement. This may take up to 6 weeks. A milk-free diet should only ever be started under medical and dietetic supervision.

5. Unknown

If dietary change, inadequate fluid intake and incorrect feed preparation have been excluded as causes of constipation and it continues to be a problem, some simple age-appropriate measures can be tried. As constipation is very often only a temporary problem, you should not need to continue these measures for long.

diluted fruit juice

- To prepare 60 mls of diluted apple or pear juice for babies less than 6 months old add 45 mls cooled boiled water to 15 mls juice (1 part juice to 3 parts water).
- To prepare 120 mls diluted apple or pear juice for babies of 6 months or older add 60 mls freshly drawn water to 60 mls juice (1 part juice to 1 part water).

Juice should only be given until the constipation has been resolved.

Dietary treatment for constipation

Babies of up to 8 weeks Offer 30 mls cooled boiled water once or twice a day. If constipation fails to resolve after a couple of days, contact your GP or PHN for further advice. If your baby is less than 3 months old, is constipated and has poor weight gain, you should contact your doctor.

Babies aged 8 weeks–6 months Offer 30–60 mls cooled boiled water twice a day e.g. between the morning and evening feeds. If constipation fails to improve give diluted apple or pear juice instead of the cooled boiled water.

Bottle-fed babies of 4–6 months who are being weaned Offer stewed pear, mango, plums or apple and/or puréed vegetables.

Babies aged 6–12 months   Offer 60–120 mls freshly drawn tap water twice a day; stewed pear, plums, mango, prunes or apple once or twice a day (add to porridge, baby rice, yogurt etc.); cooked vegetables; cereals e.g. porridge (well cooked), Ready Brek or Weetabix. If the constipation fails to improve offer 60–120 mls diluted apple or pear juice twice a day.

Note Dried fruit, such as prunes and apricots can have a mild laxative effect. Dried prunes can be boiled in some water or soaked in some orange juice and pureed.

fruit juice given to babies should be
- Pasteurised
- Unsweetened
- Diluted

giving fruit juice to infants

It is normally recommended not to give fruit juice to babies who are less than 6 months old but the treatment of constipation is the exception to this rule.

When giving juice, remember:

- Undiluted fruit juice is not suitable for babies due to its high sugar and potassium content.
- Babies younger than 8 weeks should not be given juice.
- Juices offered to babies should be unsweetened and pasteurised (juice in cartons that do not need to be stored in the fridge before being opened has been pasteurised).
- Juice should only be given until the constipation has resolved.
- Offer juice from a cup if the baby is able to drink the required volume.
- Juice given as a treatment for constipation is at a much stronger concentration than that recommended for juice offered as a drink (1 part juice to 5–10 parts cooled boiled water up to 6 months, freshly drawn tap water after 6 months).
- Prune juice, including diluted prune juice, should not be given to babies under 1 year of age due to its high sugar and sorbitol content.

Cow & Gate Comfort, Aptamil Comfort or SMA Comfort

If your baby has persistent constipation consider a week's trial on Cow & Gate Comfort, Aptamil Comfort or SMA Comfort. These formulas contain a special type of fat blend which has been shown to give softer stools. A slightly bigger teat hole may be needed for these formulae.

Non dietary treatments for constipation

Laying the baby on the back and gently moving his or her legs backwards and forwards in a 'bicycle' motion can help as this puts pressure on the intestine, which can stimulate bowel movement.

Massaging the baby's tummy may also be of benefit. A baby's large bowel sits in the abdomen (the area under the ribs) in one big loop. Stool travels around the large bowel in a clockwise direction. When giving your baby a tummy massage it is best to make clockwise circular motions from the belly button outwards.

A warm bath can also help to put the baby at ease and relieve some of the tension in the bowel.

Laxatives

Laxatives are necessary if the constipation is severe or fails to respond to dietary measures. Different laxatives work in different ways. A laxative may soften the stool, or stimulate the natural contraction of the bowel, in order to push the stool out, or both soften the stool and stimulate the bowel contraction, or provide additional fibre.

If used correctly, laxatives can be very effective in treating constipation and bring great relief to the baby. However, most of the many different types of laxatives that can be bought over the counter are not suitable for babies and small children. Your doctor or pharmacist will advise what is the best treatment.

don't give bran

Unprocessed bran should not be given to infants or young children as it is too harsh on their tummies and can reduce the absorption of some important nutrients such as zinc and iron.

when to see your doctor

- If the baby cries while straining. If a baby's stool is very hard, it can cause a small tear in the anus known as an anal fissure. This can cause a lot of discomfort and pain.
- If constipation remains a persistent problem i.e. lasts longer than three weeks.
- If the constipation is severe.
- If the baby passes an unusual stool.
- If there is blood in the baby's stool.

It is natural for parents to have reservations about giving their babies medication but if laxatives are appropriately prescribed they can sometimes offer the best solution to what is usually only a temporary problem.

Reflux

Reflux occurs when small quantities of formula or breast milk are vomited soon after feeding. Vomits are usually effortless and the amount of milk lost is not large. This is known as simple gastro-oesophageal reflux (GOR) and is a very common problem affecting at least 40 per cent of babies. These babies are sometimes referred to as the 'happy spitters'!

If a baby is gaining weight and is otherwise well, there is usually nothing to worry about. Most babies grow out of this problem during the first year. It often shows signs of improvement once they start on solids.

Cause of reflux

There is a special ring of muscle at the point where the food pipe (oesophagus) joins the stomach. This ring of muscle closes the opening between the food pipe and stomach once food has been eaten. In babies this muscle can be immature and relaxes at inappropriate times allowing stomach contents to come back up the oesophagus. Even a small or very mild reflux can cause a baby to spit up milk because the infant oesophagus is quite short compared to older children and adults.

Note Babies with reflux may not vomit after every feed. It is common for reflux to occur after some feeds but not others. There may be no pattern to the reflux.

Tips to help manage reflux

- Try to reduce the baby's wind—see pages 91–3. Winding against the shoulder may be the most comfortable position.
- Discourage your baby from drinking too quickly or gulping the feed. Ensure the teat size is appropriate.
- Avoid large feeds; smaller, more frequent volumes may be better tolerated. See page 62 for a guide to age-appropriate volume and frequency of feeds.
- Sit the baby up nice and straight during feeds—place a hand under the chin and draw the baby up.
- Try to keep your baby upright after feeds for at least 30 minutes. Where possible try not to lie your baby flat—raise the mattress or head of the cot a little, for example, by placing one or two rolled-up towels underneath the head of the mattress. It should be elevated slightly at a 30 degree angle. To reduce the risk of sudden infant death syndrome, babies should always be placed on their backs on a firm surface to sleep.

Pillows should never be used and baby's feet should always be placed at the foot of the cot to ensure he or she cannot slide down under the blankets and suffocate.

▨ Don't move or jiggle your baby immediately after a feed.

▨ Avoid tight waist bands which may create extra pressure on the baby's abdomen.

▨ Avoid exposure to smoke (tobacco or other) as it causes irritability.

▨ Avoid using a car seat immediately after feeding.

▨ Place a cushion under your baby's head when changing nappies.

> **possetting**
> Babies will often bring up a small amount of milk during winding when they burp. This is called possetting and is perfectly normal.

Thickened formula

If these measures fail to reduce reflux but the baby is growing well and is otherwise happy then the best course of action is to do nothing else. However, if reflux is causing problems—if the baby needs several changes of clothes in a day and/or social outings are difficult—offering the baby a thickened formula may help. A thicker liquid settles more easily in the stomach and is harder for the baby to bring back up.

There are three ways to thicken the baby's feed:

1. Change to a pre-thickened formula such as Enfamil AR or SMA Stay down, or
2. Add a feed-thickening agent to the normal formula or give it as a paste before breast feeding, or
3. Add a surface agent to the normal formula or give it as a paste after breast feeding.

Note Use only one of these methods at a time—do not combine methods. Always check with your doctor, public health/practice nurse or dietitian before making any changes to your baby's feeds.

1. Pre-thickened formula

Enfamil AR is based on cow's milk, contains LCPs and has a similar taste to routine formula. It contains a special rice starch thickener which only thickens once it is inside the baby's stomach. When Enfamil AR is made up ready to feed it is only marginally thicker than routine formula though you may find you need a slightly bigger sized teat hole (see pages 53–4 for more information on teat size and checking the flow rate).

Once inside the stomach the rice starch in the formula reacts with stomach acid and the feed changes into a much thicker liquid. (Acid is naturally produced in the stomach. It is part of the body's defence against germs). This thicker liquid is just as easily digested as routine formula.

> **making up pre-thickened formula**
> The Food Safety Authority of Ireland recommends that baby formula powder should be made up using water at a temperature of 70°C. Where this is not possible — as in the case of pre-thickened formulas — the feeds should be freshly prepared each time just before feeding. The volume of previously boiled water needed for a day's feeds can be added to the required number of sterilised feeding bottles and stored in the fridge until needed.

Because Enfamil AR contains rice starch it has to be made up a little differently from routine formula. As we know, formula should usually be made up with water at a temperature of 70°C to destroy any bacteria that may be present but to ensure that the Enfamil AR formula powder dissolves completely and does not clog the teat, cold water must be used to make it up. You should give the feed immediately it is made up to reduce the risk of bacteria multiplying.

You will need to let boiled water cool to cold before making up the milk. It may be helpful to pour enough boiled water for a day's supply of feeds into the required number of sterilised feeding bottles and store in the fridge until needed. Once you add the powder to the water, roll the bottle between your hands first and then shake it up and down. The rolling action helps the powder to dissolve.

SMA Stay down is based on cow's milk and has a similar taste to routine formula. It contains a special pre-cooked corn-starch thickener and works in exactly the same way as Enfamil AR.

This formula should also be made up using previously boiled water that has been left cool to cold. Don't shake the bottle; instead dissolve the powder by rolling the bottle vigorously between the hands. Give the feed immediately it is made up.

Both Enfamil AR and SMA Stay down can only be bought from a pharmacist but they are not actually prescription items. This means they are not available on the medical card and their cost cannot be reclaimed under the drug payment scheme. They are slightly more expensive than routine formula and cost may vary from pharmacy to pharmacy.

Both feeds are suitable from birth up until 12 months of age.

Pre-thickened formulas may not be as effective if your baby is taking an antacid medication e.g. Rantitidine (Zantac) or Losec (Omeprazole).They should not be used with Gaviscon Infant or thickening agents such as Carobel.

2. Feed-thickening agents

An alternative to pre-thickened formulas is the addition of a thickening agent, such as Cow & Gate Instant Carobel, to regular formula or breast milk.

Carobel is a white powder containing carob bean gum and maltodextrin and comes packaged in a box similar to powdered spoon feeds. A small sterile plastic scoop is provided in the box separate from the powder. In a small number of babies the maltodextrin present in Carobel may cause diarrhoea.

For breastfed babies Carobel should be made up to form a gel using cooled boiled water. To prepare the Carobel gel take a sterilised plastic weaning spoon and mix one level scoop of Carobel with 15 mls of the water. Stir well. Leave for 3–4 minutes to thicken. Stir again. The gel should be freshly prepared before every feed in a sterilised container. You could also use expressed breast milk instead of water.

Offer the baby 1–2 teaspoons of Carobel gel from a sterilised plastic spoon before putting to the breast and again either half way through the breast feed or after changing to the second breast.

The Food Safety Authority of Ireland recommends that thickening agents such as Carobel should be prepared using water at a temperature of 70°C. Water needs to be boiled and allowed to cool for 30 minutes to reach the recommended temperature. (Boiling water can't be used as it reacts with Carobel to form clumps).

Breastfed babies feed on demand so it is not always possible to predict feeding times. To avoid having to wait 30 minutes for boiled water to cool to the appropriate temperature while your baby is crying and hungry you could boil the water in advance, cool it to the appropriate temperature and then store it in a sterilised vacuum flask.

Regardless of water temperature, or the use of expressed breast milk, Carobel gel should always be freshly prepared before every feed. Alternatively if you prefer, you can use Gaviscon Infant.

For bottle-fed babies Make up the formula in the normal way using previously boiled water cooled to 70 degrees C. Then add the recommended dose: half a level scoop of Carobel to every 3 oz or 90 mls of formula. It's best to add the Carobel at this stage, when the water is at 70 degrees C, rather than later after the formula has cooled. Shake the bottle well. It takes 3–4 minutes for the feed to thicken. Carobel will continue to thicken for up to 15 minutes after mixing. You can start cooling the milk while it is thickening. (Feeds that are being made up for use later can be placed in the fridge once cool.).

It may be necessary to widen the hole in the teat or use a teat with a bigger hole (see pages 53–4).

Always shake the feed a second time before giving it to the baby. If your baby suffers a lot with wind and it takes too long for air bubbles to settle before feeding, instead of shaking the feed it may be better to swirl for several seconds..

If the reflux does not improve you could increase the dose of Carobel to two level scoops per 4 oz or 120 mls of formula.

Note If your baby struggles to drink the thickened formula or starts to tire quickly during feeds you may need to discontinue Carobel or reduce the dose.

3. Gaviscon Infant

The third option for treating babies with reflux is to use Gaviscon Infant. Gaviscon Infant contains sodium alginate and magnesium alginate. It works by forming a surface gel over

> **carobel**
> is only available from pharmacists. It can be bought without prescription but it is GMS listed and the cost can be reclaimed under the drugs payment scheme. It is suitable from birth onwards.

the milk preventing it from going back up the oesophagus. It also helps to protect the delicate lining of the oesophagus from the stomach acid.

For breastfed babies Mix Gaviscon Infant to a paste as per the manufacturer's instructions and offer from a spoon or feeding bottle after each breast feed.

For bottle-fed babies Make up the formula in the normal way. Just before giving the feed add Gaviscon Infant to the formula as per the manufacturer's instruction.

why babies cry
Babies cry for all sorts of reasons including
- [ ] Hunger
- [ ] Overtiredness
- [ ] Mild discomfort
- [ ] Colic
- [ ] Looking for attention
- [ ] Wanting a cuddle

Note Gaviscon Infant should not be given more than 6 times in 24 hours. It is a medicine and should only be used under medical supervision. It can be bought over the counter from pharmacists but is also available on the medical card or alternatively its cost can be reclaimed under the drug payment scheme if bought using a prescription. It is safe to use Gaviscon Infant for a prolonged period of time if needed.

Discontinuing thickened feeds
Once your baby is able to sit unsupported, reflux usually starts to improve. To check if your baby still needs a thickened feed the best thing to do is give normal formula without anything added and see if your baby vomits. If vomiting is still a problem then switch back to thickened feeds and try again in a few weeks. (See Chapter 8, pages 116–17 for advice on dealing with GORD, a more serious form of reflux.)

ask for advice
If you are worried that your baby is overfeeding or you are finding the feeding routine difficult to cope with, you should ask your doctor, public health nurse or dietitian for further advice.

Overfeeding
Overfeeding is rare in breastfed babies as they usually feed to appetite and it is not possible to offer the baby a fixed volume of milk. It is unusual for a baby to take more milk than needed so overfeeding to the point of a baby actually becoming overweight or obese is uncommon (although we have seen it happen). However, sometimes a baby does not know when to stop feeding and drinks a large volume only to vomit some of it back up.

Remember that you don't need to feed your baby every time he or she cries. As a general rule a feed should not be needed within two hours of the previous one. Your baby needs time to develop a proper hunger for feeds and should not be fed every time he or she feels a little peckish. (See pages 38–9 for an approximate guide to how much and how often your baby should feed.)

Tips to reduce overfeeding in bottle-fed babies
- Let your baby feed to appetite. The bottle does not have to be finished every time—

indeed it is normal for babies to vary a little the amount of formula they take from feed to feed.

- Try using a slower teat if your baby finishes the bottle too quickly and cries for more milk. A feed should last on average 20 minutes. Some babies are fast feeders and may finish a bottle in 10 minutes. Other babies are slow feeders and may take up to an hour to finish a bottle.

- Try distracting your baby if he or she cries when a feed is over, e.g. walk around with the baby in your arms. This will allow time for the stomach to send a message to the brain, saying that it's full.

If your baby is drinking a lot of formula

Remember it is normal for your baby to feed more on some days than others, especially during a growth spurt. Weight gain is the best indicator of whether or not a baby is taking too much formula. If weight gain is normal the baby is taking the right volume of formula. If feeding is regular throughout the day e.g. every two hours it may help to offer a bigger volume at each feed.

Consider changing to a casein-based milk such as SMA Extra Hungry Infant Milk, Aptamil Hungry Milk or Cow & Gate Infant Milk for hungrier babies. However, there is no guarantee that this will make a difference.

You could also consider starting solids at 17 weeks of age. (To allow the baby's gut adequate time to mature solids should never be introduced before 17 weeks.) Solids should not be added to the baby's bottle as this will increase the risk of obesity and may be harmful to teeth.

Teething

Teething can begin as early as 4 months, although you may not see any teeth appear until the baby is 7 months old. The eruption of the teeth can be accompanied by discomfort, irritability, cheek flushing and drooling. It may even cause a marked constitutional upset e.g. runny bowel motions, disrupted sleeping and feeding patterns.

To help soothe sore gums give your baby something hard to chew on such as a clean, cool teething ring.

Teeth are never decayed when they erupt. Once teeth appear (the two bottom front teeth usually appear first) clean them daily; this is important for long-term dental health. Brush gently with a soft brush or a soft wash cloth and water only. Don't use toothpaste until the child is 2 years old as babies and small children are unable to spit it out.

babies use their gums on solids
Teeth are not essential for good nutrition during weaning as babies use their gums to chew lumpier food. Whether or not a baby has teeth has no bearing on the weaning process.

Even though the first set of teeth will fall out, tooth decay can hasten this process and leave gaps before the permanent teeth are ready to come in. The remaining primary teeth may then crowd together to attempt to fill the gaps, which may cause the permanent teeth to come in crooked and out of place.

To avoid tooth decay protect your baby's first teeth from being damaged by prolonged and frequent exposure to sweet food and drinks.

- Don't let your baby sleep with a bottle in his/her mouth.
- Give cool boiled water, not juice, when additional fluid is required.
- If juices are used choose pure fruit juice and dilute well with water (1 part juice to 5–10 parts water).
- Avoid fizzy or carbonated drinks including sparkling water.
- When the baby is older don't give him or her sweet snacks (biscuits, chocolate, and jellies) or give them sparingly.
- Don't dip a soother in honey, sugar, syrup or other sweet food.

Less common infant feeding problems

8

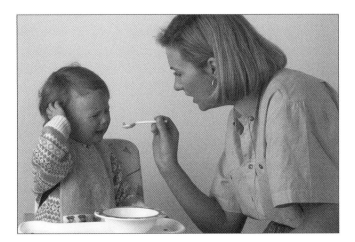

In this chapter we look at some problems that may arise in your baby's first year that cannot always be managed at home. Babies can become very ill very quickly and, although fortunately this does not happen often, if it does you need to react quickly. This is particularly important if your baby develops gastroenteritis. There is excellent treatment for these problems and your baby should quickly recover when the right approach is followed.

We also advise on how to monitor your child's growth and what to do if it falters, or your baby does not feed enough.

Lactose intolerance

Lactose is a sugar naturally present in milk, including breast milk. It is also contained in most dairy products. The enzyme that digests lactose is called lactase and is located on the surface of the gut wall. When the gut wall becomes inflamed or damaged, for example during an infection, the amount of lactase present decreases temporarily affecting the digestion of lactose.

lactose intolerance symptom and cause

- The most common symptom of temporary lactose intolerance in babies is diarrhoea; the stool is described as 'foamy' or 'frothy'.
- The most common cause of lactose intolerance in babies is gastroenteritis.

Occasionally, following a dose of diarrhoea, a baby may develop temporary lactose intolerance. Lactose levels usually return to normal within 6–8 weeks.

Undigested lactose passes through to the large bowel where gut bacteria break it down and produce gases in the process. The rapid production of these gases can cause abdominal distension and colicky pain. Occasionally, lactose intolerance can cause colic.

While lactose intolerance is not very common it should be suspected if a baby who has had gastroenteritis has persistent diarrhoea following the re-introduction of formula feeds or with breast feeding. The baby's tummy may be bloated and he or she may have crampy pain. If your baby has persistent diarrhoea, speak to your doctor.

Treatment of lactose intolerance

Lactose intolerance is easily treated by either switching to a low-lactose formula such as Enfamil O-Lac, SMA LF Lactose Free Formula or Aptamil Lactose Free, or treating the baby's normal milk (including expressed breast milk) with lactase drops such as Colief Infant Drops.

If you are breastfeeding continue as usual but in addition offer a small volume of expressed milk with Colief just before every feed. Place a few teaspoons of breast milk into a small sterilised container. Add 4 drops of Colief Infant Drops. Give this to your baby on a sterilised plastic weaning spoon just before a breast feed.

If you are bottle-feeding refer to the manufacturer's instructions regarding the addition of Colief drops to infant formula. Alternatively it may be more effective to switch to a low-lactose formula such as SMA LF Lactose Free Formula, Aptamil Lactose Free or Enfamil O-Lac. They are nutritionally complete and both contain cow's milk protein and so have the same taste and appearance as routine formula. This will make it easier for the baby to switch from the usual formula to the low-lactose milk and back again. Lactose free formulae are suitable from birth up. A trial period of 4–5 days is recommended.

A low-lactose feed will only be needed for 6–8 weeks and should only be started on the advice of your doctor, nurse, pharmacist or dietitian.

Soya infant formula is lactose free but is not recommended for babies less than 6 months old where a safe and acceptable alternative is available (for more information see Chapter 4).

It is usually quite safe to give babies of 6 months or older, who have been weaned onto solids, lactose-containing foods such as yogurt or custard.

Cow's milk protein allergy

Cow's milk allergy is estimated to affect around 2 per cent of babies. It is more common in babies fed infant formula than in exclusively breastfed babies. The good news is that 50 per cent of babies outgrow the allergy by their first birthday and this figure rises to 90 per cent by 3 years of age. For more detailed information on food allergy refer to Chapter 13.

Causes of cow's milk protein allergy

Any one of several different proteins in cow's milk can trigger an allergic reaction from the body's immune system. A baby is more likely to develop a food allergy if there is a

reintroduce regular formula gradually

When changing back from lactose-free or hypoallergenic formula to a regular formula it is best to give only a small volume of the regular formula initially e.g. mix 30 mls of regular formula with the lactose-free or hypoallergenic formula and increase the proportion of regular formula slowly over a few days.

lactase drops

Colief Infant Drops contain the enzyme lactase which is necessary for the digestion of lactose. If your baby has colic you should add these drops to expressed breast milk or infant formula to reduce the lactose content. The drops can be given to babies from birth onwards.

positive family history. In a small number of cases allergy to cow's milk can develop following a severe episode of gastroenteritis.

Infant formula does not contain the full range of these proteins as it has been extensively modified. It is for this reason that some babies have no allergy to formula milk but are allergic to ordinary cow's milk.

When babies are breastfed, cow's milk allergy, if it occurs, usually does so following the introduction of cow's milk-based infant formula. However, in a very small number of cases (about 0.5 per cent) breastfed babies react to tiny amounts of cow's milk protein present in breast milk from the mother's diet.

Symptoms of cow's milk allergy

Gastrointestinal symptoms include vomiting, diarrhoea, colic, reflux, inadequate weight gain, constipation, blood in stools. *Skin symptoms* include hives and rash. Behavioural symptoms such as irritability, crying and feed refusal may also occur.

However, not all babies with these symptoms have a cow's milk allergy and expert medical advice is always needed to confirm a diagnosis. (See Chapter 13.) Once the baby starts treatment it may take a couple of weeks before symptoms completely clear up. If your baby is started on a new formula don't worry if some symptoms continue. This can be normal and does not mean that the new formula is not working.

Treatment of cow's milk allergy

Breastfeeding You can continue breastfeeding if your baby has reacted to the tiny amounts of cow's milk protein in breast milk, but you will need to avoid milk and all milk-containing foods. Since it is very difficult for you to achieve an adequate calcium intake on a milk-free diet, and it is also difficult to completely avoid all foods containing milk, you should get expert dietary advice from a dietitian. *Note* It can take up to 2 weeks on a milk-free diet before symptoms improve.

In some very extreme cases a baby's symptoms may fail to improve despite the mother following a milk-free diet and she will need to stop breastfeeding altogether.

Breastfeeding mothers do not need to go on a milk-free diet if their baby develops a cow's milk allergy following the introduction of cow's milk formula or dairy foods into the weaning diet. In this case it should be sufficient to avoid giving the baby food containing milk and to offer a suitable infant formula such as Nutramigen 1 or Aptamil Pepti 1. Both are cow's milk based but the protein has been extensively broken down and is well tolerated.

Bottle-feeding If your baby has cow's milk allergy you will need to change the formula. The best formula for the treatment of cow's milk allergy is one with confirmed reduced allergenicity such as Nutramigen 1 or Aptamil Pepti 1. Both are cow's milk-based but the protein has been extensively broken down and is well tolerated. These formulas are available from pharmacies and can be bought without a prescription. For more detailed information about these formulas see Chapter 13.

Weaning diet You will also need to avoid giving foods containing milk in the weaning diet. Ideally you should obtain advice from an experienced paediatric dietitian to ensure that your baby's diet continues to provide the right amounts of all essential nutrients. Cutting out milk and milk-containing foods can badly affect calcium, vitamin B_{12} and protein intake but drinking a sufficient volume of a suitable infant formula will offset this.

Goat's and sheep's milk should not be used as a treatment for cow's milk allergy as they are just as allergenic as cow's milk. The proteins present in all three milks are quite similar making a cross reaction very likely. An allergic reaction to one is very likely to be followed by a reaction to the other two.

Soya protein, while completely different to cow's milk protein, can also cause allergic reactions and for this reason soya formula is generally not recommended, especially if the baby has gastrointestinal symptoms. Moreover, there have been some health concerns regarding the use of soya formula for infants less than 6 months old (see Chapter 4, page 47).

Gastroenteritis

Gastroenteritis ('gastro') is a bowel infection which causes diarrhoea (runny, watery stools) and sometimes vomiting. The vomiting may settle quickly but the diarrhoea can last for up to 10 days.

Gastro can be caused by many different germs and viruses, and is more common and severe in babies and young children under the age of 2 years. A virus known as rotavirus is the leading cause of gastro in this age group. Breastfed babies experience fewer episodes of gastroenteritis than bottle-fed babies.

It was believed for many years that children with acute diarrhoea should be starved for 24 hours in order to decrease the severity and duration of diarrhoea. However, this is now believed to be unnecessary and both the World Health Organisation (WHO) and the European Society of Paediatric Gastroenterology, Hepatology and Nutrition (ESPGHAN) recommend early feeding of infant formula or continuing breastfeeding in the management of gastroenteritis along with an oral rehydration solution.

Dehydration

Babies and young children with gastro can become very ill very quickly due to a rapid loss of body water and salts resulting in severe dehydration. Babies younger than 6 months are most at risk.

Early signs of dehydration include thirst and a mild reduction in urine output. Signs of more advanced dehydration include dry lips or mouth, not passing urine, becoming drowsy and cold hands and feet.

Weight is another useful marker of dehydration. For every 100 mls of body water lost, a baby's weight automatically drops by 100 g. (Over 60 per cent of a baby's body is made up of water).

During an episode of gastroenteritis babies under 6 months may need to be seen by their doctor every 6–12 hours. If the doctor is worried that the baby is becoming dehydrated he or she may refer the baby to hospital for closer monitoring. Gastro is one of the commonest reasons for admission to hospital for children under 5 years.

signs of dehydration

Always bring your baby to the GP or hospital as quickly as possible if there are any signs of dehydration.

Early signs
- Thirst
- Mild reduction in number of wet nappies

More advanced dehydration
- Dry lips or mouth
- Drowsiness or sunken eyes
- Not passing urine
- Refusal to drink formula or other fluids for more than 6 hours
- Vomiting replacement fluid
- Cold hands and feet

Medications

Do not give medicines to reduce the vomiting and diarrhoea. These are not of benefit and may actually be harmful.

Treatment of mild gastroenteritis

Babies and children with mild gastro can be looked after at home. The main treatment is to prevent dehydration by replacing fluid lost from diarrhoea and/or vomiting. Therefore it is vitally important for the baby to drink fluids. Fluids should be taken even if the diarrhoea seems to get worse.

If the baby is vomiting, small amounts of fluid should be given often e.g. using a teaspoon. The best type of fluid to give is an oral rehydration solution.

Oral rehydration solutions (ORS)

Oral rehydration solutions are life saving and represent one of the most important advances in modern medicine since the discovery of antibiotics. They are used to manage diarrhoea in both children and adults. ORS should be initiated as soon as diarrhoea starts in order to prevent or correct dehydration.

Watery diarrhoea contains a lot of sodium which has been lost from the body. To replace this loss oral rehydration solutions contain almost 10 times the level of sodium found in baby milk formulas and also have some extra potassium. A small amount of sugar (2 g per 100 mls) is present in ORS and this special combination of sugar and sodium works a kind of magic on the gut, making it absorb water more easily.

The two main brands available in Ireland are Dioralyte and Rapolyte. They come in powdered sachets and are prepared by dissolving the powder in freshly cooled boiled water as per the manufacturers' instructions. Both neutral and flavoured varieties are available. For babies the neutral variety is preferable so as not to encourage a sweet tooth.

It is not a good idea to give carbonated drinks such as 7-Up as a form of treatment for gastro in babies. Although 7-Up does contain sodium, the sodium and sugar are not present in the right amounts and so cannot match the rehydration provided by ORS. Indeed the high level of sugar in 7-Up (11 g per 100 mls) may make the diarrhoea worse. Diet 7-Up is even more unsuitable as it does not contain any sugar at all.

Handwashing

Your baby or child is infectious so wash your hands well with soap and warm water, particularly before feeding and after changing nappies. Gastro is very easily spread. Virus particles are shed in the vomit and diarrhoea, and are transferred from one person to another through close contact e.g. sharing food, water and eating utensils, and the particles can also be transmitted in the air.

Treating breastfed babies with gastroenteritis

- Continue breastfeeds, stop solids.
- Offer ORS after feeds every time a diarrhoeal stool is passed. Try to get the baby to take 30–90 mls (1–3 oz) depending on size (10 mls for every kilo).
- If ORS is tolerated, re-introduce solids after 4 hours once the baby is re-hydrated.
- Offer supplements of ORS for as long as the baby continues to have diarrhoea.

Note The positive effect of continuing breastfeeding along with offering ORS supplements during gastroenteritis is well established.

Treating bottle-fed babies with gastroenteritis

- Stop milk feeds and stop solids.
- Offer ORS instead of milk feeds.
- If ORS is tolerated i.e. is not vomited back up and the diarrhoea does not get worse, after 4 hours reintroduce normal full-strength formula.
- Formula should not be stopped for more than 12–24 hours.
- If formula is tolerated, reintroduce solids.
- Continue to offer ORS supplements between or after feeds for as long as the baby has diarrhoea. This will help replace fluid and salt losses.

- Repeated projectile (forceful) vomiting
- Poor weight gain
- Feed refusal or pain on feeding
- Inconsolable crying
- Regurgitation of blood
- Respiratory symptoms e.g. apnoea (temporary stoppage of breathing)

There are a number of very serious medical conditions besides GORD that may present with some of the above symptoms. A thorough examination by a doctor is essential to rule out any other underlying causes and to ensure prompt medical treatment where necessary.

effects of faltering growth

Medical research in the area of infant nutrition has made some very important discoveries over the last number of years. It is now known that sub-optimal nutrition during the first two years of life can have far reaching consequences. Nutrition from the time of conception to 2 years of age influences lifelong health, including the onset of diseases such as diabetes, coronary heart disease and high blood pressure.

Signs that your baby may need to be admitted to hospital

- Dehydration: dry mouth, sunken eyes or drowsiness.
- No wet nappy for more than 6 hours.
- Vomiting the ORS solution.
- Refusal to drink fluids.
- Diarrhoea lasting longer than 2 weeks.

If your baby has any of these symptoms you should bring him or her to your GP who will assess your baby and advise you accordingly.

Gastro-oesophageal reflux disease (GORD)

Gastro-oesophageal reflux disease (GORD) is a severe form of reflux. Babies can have projectile vomits and weight loss. They may be irritable during feeds and refuse to drink more than a few ounces of feed at a time.

Parents often report that their baby is hungry for feeds, feeds well at the beginning of the feed but stops after only taking a couple of ounces.

Sometimes babies with GORD are very distressed and cry inconsolably for long periods at any time during the day or night. In a small number of cases babies with GORD have 'silent' reflux and do not have any vomits.

If your baby has any of these symptoms you should get advice from your GP without delay. Your doctor may suggest a trial of Gaviscon Infant for 2–3 days. However, this many not help babies with severe reflux.

Babies with severe reflux often have oesophagitis which is inflammation of the food pipe caused by repeated contact with stomach acid. Babies with reflux oesophagitis sometimes arch their backs in pain during feeding and their whole body may become rigid.

Your doctor may prescribe a medication to reduce stomach acid production such as Ranitidine or Zantac. This medication can give the baby great relief and a dramatic improvement is usually seen within 72 hours.

Babies may also require thickened feeds (see pages 103–4) as part of their treatment. However, the pre-thickened formulas Enfamil AR and SMA Stay down may not be effective for babies on acid-reducing medication.

In a small number of cases GORD may be caused by a cow's milk protein allergy. If the reflux fails to respond to treatment then a 1–2 week trial on a hypoallergenic formula such as Nutramigen or Aptamil Pepti should be considered. Breastfeeding mothers should consider a week's trial on a dairy-free diet but this should only be done under a dietician's supervision. For additional information and support refer to the excellent website www.livingwithreflux.org.

Faltering growth

Faltering growth is not a specific disease but rather an observation of poor growth. During the first year of life an infant grows more rapidly than at any other time of life (or at least life outside the womb). The baby's weight gain is the best indication as to whether feeding is adequate and development is proceeding as it should. Faltering growth occurs when an infant's rate of growth fails to meet the potential expected for age.

Prolonged faltering growth must be prevented as it causes developmental delay due to poor brain growth and short stature.

Normal weight gain in the first year of life

Remember that all babies are different and may have a variable weight gain, gaining a lot of weight one week and not so much the next. While it is important that a baby gains weight steadily, a week or two gaining slightly more or less weight than ideal does no harm. The following is a guide to your baby's expected weight gain during the first year.

Expected weight gain during the first year of life	
Age	Weekly weight gain
0–3 months	180–285g
4–6 months	90–140g
7–9 months	55–80g
10–12 months	40–60g

Naturally small babies usually gain less weight per week compared to bigger babies of the same age. It is normal for some naturally small breastfed babies to gain only 125 g per week during the first 3 months.

Babies grow on average 2 cm a month or 25 cm in the first year, and double in length by the first birthday. (A child's height at age 2 is roughly half eventual adult height.)

Expected growth in height/length during the first 12 months

A baby grows on average 2 cm per month, or 25 cm in the first year, and doubles in length by the first birthday. (By 2 years of age a child is roughly half the eventual adult height.)

Expected head circumference growth rate during the first 12 months

Head circumference is a measure of the baby's head size and this is a reflection of brain growth. Brain growth during the first year is incredibly rapid—1 cm per month. By the baby's second birthday the brain will have grown to reach 80 per cent of its adult size.

What are growth charts?

Growth charts are a series of curves used to compare an infant's growth to that of other healthy infants of the same age. They are also a very useful tool for monitoring an infant's growth over time. Growth charts are used by doctors, nurses and dietitians. (See pages 8 and 10 of your baby's Child Health Record booklet for a basic growth chart.)

A baby's position on the curve is referred to as his or her centile position. As a baby grows, weight, length and head circumference usually, though not always, track along a particular centile. Birth weight may not reflect a baby's 'true' centile position as it is influenced more by the mother's diet and the efficiency of the placenta than genetic factors. It is normal for some babies to be bigger than average and some smaller.

Breastfed babies have a different rate of growth to bottle-fed babies, gaining slightly more weight during the first 3 months and having a slightly slower weight gain thereafter. This is the optimal rate of growth for all babies whether they are breastfed or bottle-fed. Babies born in Ireland after 1 January 2013 should have their growth plotted on the UK-WHO-Ireland Growth charts. These charts are based on the growth rates of healthy breastfed babies.

How often should I weigh my baby?

A healthy full-term baby should not be weighed more than once a week. Weighing scales are not always accurate and different scales may give slightly different weights. Ideally babies should always be weighed at the same time of day, naked and on the same weighing scales.

Weighing a baby before or after a feed or wet nappy affects their weight! For example, a baby who is weighed just after drinking a 120 mls bottle will weigh 120 g more than they actually are. If you are concerned about your baby's weight it is best to speak to your GP, nurse or dietitian.

Causes of faltering growth

In infancy growth is chiefly controlled by nutrition. Fewer than 5 per cent of children with faltering growth are found to have something medically wrong with them.

when to measure your baby's growth during the first 12 months

Growth is a key indicator of normal health and development. Ideally weight, length and head circumference should be checked as follows during the first year.

Age	Check
At birth	Weight and length
24–30 hours	Head circumference
10–14 days	Length (if not measured at birth), head circumference
6–8 weeks	Weight, head circumference
12 weeks	Weight and length
16 weeks	Weight
6–8 months	Weight and length
12–15 months	Weight and length

You should be able to pop into your local health centre to get your baby measured. Or check with your public health nurse or practice nurse about other options available to you.

Common causes of faltering growth

▪ Poor feeding e.g. as a result of difficulty sucking, swallowing.

▪ Poor retention of food e.g. vomiting as a result of gastro-oesophageal reflux disease (GORD).

▪ Inadequate dietary intake. It's a good idea always to make up a little more formula than you think your baby will take. This will allow the baby to stop feeding when full rather than having to stop because there is no more formula in the bottle.

▪ Acute gastrointestinal infection.

▪ Cow's milk protein allergy.

▪ Breastfeeding problem.

▪ Inappropriate weaning diet.

Treatment of faltering growth

Treatment of faltering growth depends on the cause. Regular monitoring of the baby's growth after treatment has been initiated is essential. This is important to ensure that the baby's weight and length catch up with where they should be to fulfill potential.

case history: 8-month-old Sean

Sean is taking 3 spoon feeds a day and has a good appetite for them. His diet is varied but he seems to be off his bottles and it is a struggle to get him to drink his milk. He prefers to drink some water from a beaker at mealtimes.

Is there a danger Sean will become dehydrated?
To check if Sean is becoming dehydrated count the number of wet nappies he has in a day. If there are 4 or more, and Sean is not constipated then he is taking enough fluids to maintain hydration. Dark or foul smelling urine is a sign of dehydration.

Is Sean growing well and gaining enough weight?
Ask the public health nurse to check Sean's weight and length. If he is growing well then he is getting enough calories and protein in his diet.

Is Sean getting enough calcium?
Ideally Sean should be drinking 500–600 mls of formula milk a day. However, a good compromise is to try to get him to drink a minimum of 300 mls of formula milk a day and add formula to his solids where possible. If it is not possible to add very much formula to his solids offer him milky foods such as custard, yogurt, rice pudding and cheese twice a day. It is also a good idea to change his formula to a follow-on milk which contains extra calcium, protein and iron.

Underfeeding

Most babies have an inbuilt survival instinct and will take as much milk as they need. However, some babies are not great feeders and may sleep for long periods. They don't seem hungry but are quite happy and contented in themselves.

If your baby is not taking as much milk as other babies of the same age but is gaining enough weight then there is nothing to worry about. If, however, the weight gain is not as good as it should be you will need to try to get your baby to take more milk. See Chapter 5, page 62 for a guide on how much and how often a bottle-fed baby should feed. For breastfed babies see Chapter 3, pages 38–9.

Some tips to help your baby feed better

- If your baby is falling asleep during feeds, try gently pressing the jaw or stroking the cheeks. This can stimulate the suck and more feed will be taken.
- A nappy change half way through the feed may help to wake the baby.
- Wake the baby at least every 4 hours during the day to offer feeds.
- Try feeding in a slightly cooler room or dress the baby in fewer clothes during a feed.
- If you are bottle-feeding make sure the teat hole size suits the baby.
- A change in formula can sometimes lead to feed refusal. If the new formula has not been recommended for a specific medical reason consider going back onto the old

formula or try mixing some new formula with old formula. Slowly increasing the volume of new formula over a number of days can help the baby adjust to a new taste.

■ Ask your doctor to check your baby for any subtle signs of sucking or swallowing difficulties.

When to see your doctor

■ If your baby suddenly goes off feeds for no apparent reason and/or is irritable or crying. This can be a sign of a more serious medical problem and you should seek medical advice as soon as possible.

■ If your baby has a temporary nasal obstruction due to a chest infection. This commonly interferes with feeding and your doctor may prescribe a short course of decongestant nose drops.

■ If your baby shows signs of dehydration e.g. a reduced number of wet nappies or very dark smelly urine.

■ If your baby is not gaining enough weight.

off days are normal

It is normal for a baby to have an off day. One or two days of reduced formula intake need not be anything to worry about provided the baby seems otherwise well and has a wet nappy at least every 6 hours.

9 Healthy eating for toddlers

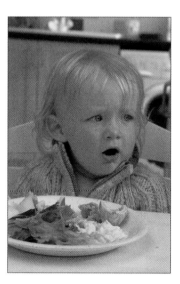

Feeding toddlers and young children can be a challenge. While their nutritional needs are still high in proportion to their body size, there are now a number of barriers to achieving a good nutritional intake that can be hard to overcome. No longer content to sit in the high chair while you spoon feed their dinners, toddlers are active and want to be a part of everything that is going on around them.

Your child may now have a very clear idea as to what he or she does or does not want to eat. This is the time when fussy eating often becomes an issue and while for most children it is just a passing phase, it can develop into a greater problem. This is also the age when a lot of children start daycare and as a result of mixing with other children, are suddenly exposed to colds and bugs that can cause tummy upsets. In this chapter we advise on how to achieve a healthy balanced diet for your toddler.

The food pyramid

Achieving a balanced diet is all about eating a variety of foods, in the right proportions, providing a good combination of protein, carbohydrate, fat, vitamins and minerals.

It is easier to achieve a balanced diet when you think of food in terms of groups rather than individual foods, for example, starchy foods or dairy foods. The food pyramid divides food into food groups and indicates how many servings of each group should be eaten each day. It is based on World Health Organisation recommendations.

The foods near the bottom of the pyramid are the ones of which most should be eaten, and the foods towards the top of the pyramid should be eaten less. The foods at the very tip of the pyramid should be eaten only on occasion. The Department of Health launched an updated Food Pyramid in December 2016. The new Food Pyramid is for adults, teenagers and children aged five and over. Updated healthy eating guidelines for children aged 1–5 are awaited.

Food pyramid Food groups & recommended portions		
Group 5 **Fizzy drinks, sweets** etc.:	eat **sparingly**	
Group 4 **Protein** Meat, chicken, peas, beans, fish:	eat **2 portions** a day	
Group 3 **Dairy products** Milk, cheese and yogurt:	eat **3 portions** a day	
Group 2 **Fruit & vegetables** Fruit, fruit juice, vegetables:	eat **2–4 portions** a day	
Group 1 **Starches** Bread, cereals, potatoes, rice and pasta:	eat **4–6 portions** a day	

Group 1 Starchy foods, including bread, potatoes, pasta, rice, breakfast cereal, crackers and other grains

The main role of starchy foods is to provide energy. The brain runs mainly on glucose as a fuel, as does muscle, and this is largely supplied in the diet by starchy foods. Starchy foods will also give your child the energy needed to run around and to concentrate on various tasks. They can also contain B vitamins, certain minerals such as calcium, iron and zinc, and some protein. Breakfast cereals generally also have added vitamins and minerals.

It is good to provide your child with some whole meal starchy foods such as brown bread or a high-fibre cereal. This can help keep the bowels working properly. Also, wholegrain bread contains iron. However, don't give your child too much whole meal or wholegrain starchy foods as too much fibre is not good for small children. It can displace other nutrients from the diet and can affect the absorption of certain nutrients.

Group 2 Fruit and vegetables, including fruit, vegetables, vegetable soup, salad vegetables, beans, tinned fruit and fruit juice

Fruit and vegetables provide your child with vitamins, minerals, antioxidants and fibre. Most fruit and vegetables are made up of water, sugar and starch and therefore also provide some energy. Fruit is naturally sweet and may satisfy a sweet craving thereby avoiding confectionery. The fibre in fruit and vegetables can help keep your child's gut healthy and can also prevent constipation. The vitamins and minerals provided by fruit and vegetables may give the immune system a boost and will keep your child looking and feeling healthy. An adequate intake of fruit and vegetables is vital for overall good health.

tips to increase vegetables in your child's diet

- Add extra vegetables to stews and casseroles e.g. turnip, celery, parsnip, or butternut squash.
- Add extra vegetables to curries e.g. mange tout or baby sweetcorn.
- Top pizza with lots of vegetables e.g. tomatoes, mushrooms, onion, sweetcorn.
- Grate carrot into bolognese sauce, making it more or less undetectable!
- Mash broccoli or another vegetable into mashed potato, again to make it less detectable.
- A number of vegetables can be used in homemade soup, then liquidised to make it more appealing. Children don't tend to like whole vegetables floating around in a soup but will happily eat soup with well-blended vegetables.
- Add vegetables to sandwiches e.g. sliced cucumber, cherry tomatoes, lettuce, scallions, celery.
- Get your child involved in preparing salads and vegetables. He or she will then be much more likely to eat them.
- Children tend to prefer crunchy vegetables to mushy ones. Try sticks of raw vegetables (peppers, carrots, celery) with a dip such as cream cheese or hummus. Try steaming green vegetables lightly until they are crunchy and drizzling a little garlic butter over them
- Try making guacamole with avocado.

tips to increase fruit in your child's diet

- Try making fruit kebabs by threading a number of tasty fruit chunks onto a skewer (e.g. fresh pineapple, banana, strawberry and pear). Brush with honey or maple syrup and place under a grill for a few minutes.
- Make a fruit smoothie. Chill the ingredients. It is good to add yogurt to the smoothies for extra calcium and protein. The smoothie should be drunk as soon as possible after it is made in order to preserve the vitamins. Frozen berries can be used in smoothies—they are less expensive.
- Add a chopped banana or a handful of raisins to your child's breakfast cereal.
- Handy fruit snacks include a small box of raisins, a mandarin, plums, cherries. These can be brought in the car for journeys.
- Have a fruit bowl stocked and within easy access so the family can snack on fruit, e.g. between meals or while watching TV, rather than on junk foods.
- Have fruit in the car for long journeys so they can choose to eat fruit themselves.
- Add fruit into pancakes and desserts or serve fresh fruit and ice-cream.
- Frozen grapes are a delicious alternative to confectionery.
- Stewed fruit is also a good dessert option, e.g. stewed apple and custard.

to preserve antioxidant levels

- Avoid overcooking vegetables; steam them or cook in a small amount of water for as short a time as possible so that they are still crisp
- Avoid soaking vegetables in water.
- Serve raw vegetables where possible.
- Cook potatoes unpeeled.
- Store salad vegetables in the refrigerator to help keep them fresh and crisp for longer.
- If storing cut vegetables or fruit place in an airtight container and refrigerate. Don't store vegetables in water as the vitamins can dissolve into the water and be lost.

Group 3 Dairy produce, including milk, cheese and yogurt

Dairy produce provide your child with calcium and protein. Adequate calcium intake is important for healthy bones, particularly for children, whose skeleton is growing. Up to 90 per cent of 'peak bone mass' is reached at 18–20 years old. Peak bone mass is the point at which the skeleton is finished growing and is the strongest it will be for adult life. If adequate calcium hasn't been provided up to that point, bones won't be as strong as they should be and osteoporosis may be a problem in later life.

Milk, cheese and yogurt are also an excellent source of protein, needed for growth and many other functions that keep the body working properly.

Dairy products contain vitamins A and B_{12} and other B vitamins. They are also a good source of zinc which may help to keep your child's immune system healthy.

Milk, breast or formula, is the main part of a child's diet for the first year of life. After that, cow's milk can become the main drink. Cow's milk contains protein, calcium and vitamins and is an important part of your child's diet. It contains fewer vitamins and minerals than formula or breast milk but by the age of 12 months, your child should be eating a varied diet with fruit and vegetables, meat, eggs, dairy products, fish, cereals and bread—the combination of all these foods with milk provides all the nutrients needed.

Dairy products get a lot of bad press these days and it is quite trendy to cut them out of the diet. However, there is no sound medical or scientific basis for this bias against dairy produce. Dietitians and health professionals totally disagree with the removal of dairy products from the diet unless it is for a specific medical reason diagnosed by a properly qualified doctor in a hospital or GP service.

There is absolutely no scientific evidence that dairy produce are mucus-producing. If you suspect that your child has a genuine allergy to dairy produce ensure that you get a proper diagnosis from a fully qualified doctor in a hospital or GP service (see also Chapter 13 on allergy). Withdrawing milk from a child's diet without need, and without the advice of a properly qualified dietitian, can lead to serious nutritional deficiencies.

Group 4 Protein foods, including meat, fish, eggs, pulses (peas, beans and lentils) and meat substitutes such as quorn and TVP

Protein foods do mainly what the name suggests, provide us with protein. Protein is needed for just about every cell in our bodies. Muscles and skin are made of protein, as are antibodies that attack bacteria and viruses. Our bodies take the protein from our diets and use it to make other proteins in the body, such as muscle.

Many foods contain protein but the foods on this shelf of the food pyramid contain a large amount of protein. Dairy products contain almost as much protein but they are kept on the shelf below as they are needed also for their calcium.

Meat, fish, eggs and pulses also contain many other important nutrients such as iron, zinc, vitamin B_{12}, vitamin D, other B vitamins and essential fats. The foods on this shelf are highly nutritious.

Group 5 The top shelf — the not-so-healthy foods, including confectionery, fizzy drinks, crisps, cakes, take-aways etc.

These foods are 'treats' only and should be used sparingly. In other words, they should only be given on occasion. It is difficult to say how often you can give these foods to children as it depends on the child but as seldom as you can is a good guideline to work with.

Recommended daily portions of each food group

	1–3 years	3–5 years
Starch	**4 portions**	**4–6+ portions**
Bread	½–1 slice	1 small slice
Cereal	1–2 tablespoons	2–3 tablespoons
Weetabix	½–1	1–1½
Potatoes, mashed	½–1 scoop	1–1½ scoops
Potatoes, boiled	½–1 potato	1–1½ potatoes
Cooked rice or pasta	1–2 tablespoons	2–3 tablespoons
Fruit and vegetables	**2–4 portions**	**4+ portions**
Apple/pear/banana	½ fruit	1 small fruit
Plum/kiwi/mandarin	½–1 fruit	1 fruit
Grapes	6–8	12
Strawberries	4	6
Tinned fruit	1 tablespoon	2 tablespoons
Carrots	½ carrot (1 tablespoon)	1 small carrot (2 tablespoons)
Other vegetables	1 tablespoon, cooked	2 tablespoons, cooked
Salad vegetables	2 tablespoons	3 tablespoons
Tomato	2 cherry/ ½ tomato	3 cherry/1 small tomato
Vegetable soup	1 small bowl	1 bowl
Dairy	**3 portions**	**3 portions**
Cheese	30 g in cubes or grated (about the size of a matchbox)	
Milk	200 ml	200 ml
Yogurt	1 pot (125 g)	1 pot (125 g)
Protein	**2 portions**	**2 portions**
Minced meat	1–1½ tablespoons	2–3 tablespoons
Meat	½–1 slice	1–2 slices
Fish fillet	¼–½ small fillet	½–1 small fillet
Fish fingers /sausages	1–2	2–3
Eggs	½–1 egg	1
Beans/lentils	1–2 tablespoons	2–3 tablespoons
Quorn/TVP	30–60g	60 g
Smooth peanut butter	1–2 tablespoons	2 tablespoons
Fatty and sugary foods	**Sparingly**	**Sparingly**
Sweets, crisps, fizzy drinks, biscuits, cakes, confectionary, take-aways, fried foods.	Occasionally	Occasionally

How much of each food group should my child be eating?

By the age of 12 months your baby should have started to eat almost the same foods as the rest of the family. Portion sizes will vary depending on your child's age, weight, and activity levels. Younger children need fewer calories per day than older children and this is reflected in their portion sizes. Let your child's appetite and weight gain at this stage be your best guide.

See the portion size guide on the previous page plus the suggested number of portions 1–3-year-olds and 3–5-year-olds need each day from the different food groups. Try to include the suggested number of portions from each food group in your child's diet each day.

Processed foods

Try to give your child plain, unprocessed meat and fish as much as possible, for example, chicken breasts, fish fillets, minced meat, pork chops. All these foods contain far less fat and salt than processed foods and are far higher in nutrients.

Processed, pre-prepared foods such as frozen pizza, frozen chips, frozen burgers, sausages, ready-made noodles, fish fingers, chicken nuggets and ready-made meals, tend to be high in salt and fat and lower in protein, vitamins and minerals. Unfortunately, they also tend to be a big hit with children.

Fresh, unprocessed food is also good for your child's taste buds as he or she learns to appreciate the real taste of meat and fish without the extra breadcrumbs and salt. If your child is constantly eating processed foods, there is little chance of developing a taste for anything else.

Obviously, there is nothing wrong with serving something like sausages and chips from time to time, even once a week, on a Saturday for example, but try to avoid giving it any more frequently than that.

processed v. unprocessed foods

- **1 small fillet of plaice (100 g)** contains 19 g protein, 2 g fat, 93 calories and 0.3 g salt.
- **3 fish fingers (84 g)** contain 12 g protein, 7 g fat, 168 calories and 0.8 g salt.

So the plaice contains far more protein and far less fat, salt and calories than the fish fingers. (1½ times more protein, less than one third of the fat, almost half the calories and almost one third of the salt.)

Simple nutritious dinners

Simple and nutritious, unprocessed dinners you can make at home for your toddler include:

- Minced meat mashed up with potato and peas
- Beef casserole or stew
- Baked fish in a white sauce with mashed potato
- Chicken curry
- Shepherd's pie
- Spaghetti bolognese (home-made)
- Fish cake

- Risotto
- Pasta and tuna bake
- Home-made burgers

Some of these dishes can be made beforehand and frozen for future use. If you are in a hurry and want to make something quickly, the following quick meals are unprocessed and very nutritious:

- Omelette
- Scrambled eggs on toast
- Beans on toast
- Cheese on toast
- Toasted sandwiches
- Baked potato done in the microwave with a cheese topping

Salt

Diets high in salt have been associated with an increased risk of high blood pressure in adults which in turn increases the risk of heart disease. The Food Safety Authority of Ireland (FSAI) recommends a maximum intake of salt of 2 g a day for 1–3 year olds and 3 g a day for 4–6 year olds. Don't add salt to your child's food as many foods already contain hidden amounts of salt.

Processed foods, especially meats, tend to be highest in salt. The label will specify how much salt is in the food.

Meal patterns and snacks

Your child should now be taking about 3 meals and 2–3 snacks per day. Snacks are an important part of your toddler's diet, helping to meet energy needs for growth.

Snack ideas for 1–5 year olds

Snacks should be just filling enough to tide your child over until the next meal but not heavy enough to ruin the appetite completely. Nutritious snacks include:

- Some raisins and a glass of milk
- Cheese cubes or triangles
- Banana
- Pineapple chunks/handful of seedless grapes
- Raw vegetable sticks with cream cheese

toddlers vary the amount they eat

A lot of parents feel that their toddler is eating very little but if you add up everything eaten over a few days you may well find that your child is eating plenty of food. Many toddlers do not eat consistent amounts of food day in, day out. They may eat very little some days and quite a lot other days — this is normal. An 'up and down' pattern of eating is nothing to worry about and tends to balance itself out over time. If your child is growing and gaining weight, he or she is obviously getting enough calories.

- Yogurt
- Sliced apple with cheese
- A small glass of smoothie made with natural yogurt
- Small bowl of cereal
- Currant bun or fruit scone
- Wholemeal bread/toast

Are there any foods I should avoid giving my toddler?

Don't give whole or chopped nuts or popcorn because of the risk of choking.

Shark, marlin and swordfish should be avoided because of the high levels of mercury these fish contain. Fresh tuna should not be given more than once a week for the same reason and tinned tuna more than twice a week.

Don't give raw eggs or any food containing raw or partially cooked eggs due to a risk of salmonella.

Do I need to give my toddler a vitamin supplement?

If your child is eating a balanced diet that includes all the major food groups a vitamin supplement will not be needed.

Exceptions to this are children on vegetarian, or otherwise limited, diets and toddlers at risk of a vitamin D deficiency (because their skin is very dark or they have little exposure to sunlight). These children may need to take a vitamin supplement and to continue on these vitamins until they are 5 years of age.

You should seek advice from your pharmacist as to which supplement to give. One recommended vitamin supplement is Abidec Multivitamin drops which contains vitamin A, some B group vitamins, vitamin C and vitamin D.

Day care

Parents are always concerned about the food their child is being given in childcare, especially if they are there for most of the day. The Health Promotion Unit of the Department of Health and Children has produced a set of guidelines 'Food and nutrition guidelines for pre-school services' which are available to download from the internet at www.dohc.ie/publications/preschool_guidelines.html.

These guidelines recommend that:

- Children in full day care (more than 5 hours) should be offered at least 2 meals, one of which should be hot, and 2 snacks. A third meal may have to be provided if children remain for a long day.
- Children in day care for a maximum of 5 hours should receive at least 2 meals and 1

snack. It is not necessary that a hot meal be provided but the main meal should include at least one serving from each of the shelves of the food pyramid.

- Children who are in day care for up to 3½ hours should be offered 1 meal and 1 snack, for example, a snack and lunch.

The key recommendations from the guidelines are as follows:
- Offer a wide variety of foods.
- Offer suitable sized portions.
- Offer healthy food choices and tooth-friendly drinks frequently.
- Accommodate special food needs of individual children.
- Plan healthy, varied meals and snacks.
- Help children learn to eat.
- Foster good dental health.
- Prepare food in a clean and safe way.
- Develop a healthy eating policy.

Illness and childcare

When children first attend day care they often pick up colds, stomach bugs and other minor illnesses from other children, especially if this is the first time they are exposed to other children. It is estimated that children attending day care have a 1½–3 times higher risk of contracting gastrointestinal and respiratory tract infections than children cared for at home or in small family care groups. Your toddler's immune system is still developing and unfortunately colds and stomach bugs are par for the course.

It is also interesting to note, however, that a number of studies have shown that children aged less than 12 months who attend day care are less likely to develop asthma and other allergic diseases. It may be useful to give your child attending day care a probiotic every day. See page 9 for more information on probiotics.

10 Shopping wisely

The supermarket can be a confusing place when you are trying to shop for healthy foods for your child. We all know that fresh fruit and vegetables are good for children as are fresh meat and fish but after that things are less clear. Media discussion about unhealthy levels of fat, sugar and salt in foods and warnings about genetically modified (GM) foods, additives and preservatives often just add to the confusion.

In this chapter we set out the latest information on what you should and should not be concerned about when shopping for food. Here you will find the knowledge and tools, especially how to assess the information given in product labels, to help you to decide which foods to buy for your child.

The power of marketing

Nutrition is big business for food manufacturers. The children's food industry, in particular, is a multi-billion dollar business. Parents want to provide their children with healthy diets but are being manipulated by clever marketing from food companies and by their children who are themselves being targeted by marketing.

Companies are constantly trying to come up with new ways to attract both children and parents to their products. They are very clued in to the role children have in persuading parents to buy them foods that appeal to them. This is known in the industry as 'pester power'. A study commissioned by the UK Food Standards Agency looked at television advertising of foods directed to children. It found that such advertising has a definite effect on children's food preferences, what their parents buy and what the children eat. The study also found that there was large-scale marketing of foods aimed at children, and that those foods were high in fat, sugar and salt.

Health professionals have been campaigning to ban the advertising of unhealthy food to children. Research carried out in 20 European countries from May to November 2004 looked at the quantity and type of advertising of unhealthy foods to children. The co-coordinators of the research found it hard to define an 'unhealthy' food as such because not all foods high in fat or sugar are unhealthy. For example, an avocado has more fat than a full-sized chocolate bar but it is still a healthier choice.

Different countries came up with different definitions of 'unhealthy' such as 'high in fat, sugar or salt'. Generally, the unhealthy foods most

The National Children's Food Survey

(Irish Universities Nutrition Alliance 2005) found that 68 per cent of parents in Ireland find it hard, at least sometimes, to provide a healthy diet to their children. The biggest problem encountered was the child's own likes and dislikes. Parents also found food and drink advertising interfered with their attempts to provide a healthy diet to their children.

frequently marketed were snacks, fast foods, confectionary, sweetened cereals and soft drinks. These foods tend to be high in fat, sugar and salt.

The research found that companies were spending considerable amounts of money marketing unhealthy foods to children. The report also noted that nearly 100 per cent of food advertising on TV aimed at children in Denmark and the UK was for unhealthy food.

Television was not the only medium used by companies to advertise to children. The internet and sponsorship of sporting or school-based events were also used.

There is no doubt that advertising is in some way contributing to the problem of obesity in Ireland with 1 in 5 children overweight or obese. According to the World Health Organisation the aggressive marketing of food (and drinks) high in fat, sugar or salt to young children could increase their risk of becoming obese (WHO 2003).

Parents are also being targeted. Food companies are very aware that parents are concerned about their children's diets and wish to provide them with the best they can. Many advertisements play up one 'healthy' side to a food, such as added calcium or vitamins, and completely downplay the fact that that particular food is packed full of sugar.

Parents are also made to feel guilty by advertising which suggests that certain products can offer benefits, for example improved immunity, to their children and that if they don't buy them they are effectively leaving their children open to infection. Parents are very vulnerable to this kind of advertising.

read the label
Only by reading labels and checking ingredients can parents get a good idea of which food products are best for their child.

How to decide if a food is healthy or not

Deciding whether a food is healthy or not is not the easiest thing in the world as the authors of the report above discovered. There is no magic formula that will distinguish between healthy and unhealthy foods. But by reading labels with nutritional information and lists of ingredients, and comparing brands you will be in a position to decide if what you are planning to buy is healthy or not.

Nutritional information on labels

Almost all foods now have a label with nutritional information such as how much sugar, fat, protein and calories are in the food. European law states that if a manufacturer makes a health claim, for example that a food is '95 per cent fat free', then it must provide a label with nutritional information. However, if no nutritional claims are made, then there is no legal obligation to provide nutritional information.

All nutrients must be given per 100 g or 100 ml of the food or drink. Manufacturers do not have to state the values per portion of the food or drink but many do.

For example, the label below gives information about energy, protein, carbohydrate, sugars, fat, saturated fat, fibre and sodium per 100 g. It also states that an average serving size is 100g and that the pack contains 2 x 100 g servings.

Typical composition	1 serving of 100 g (3½ oz) provides
Energy	1448 kJ/341 kcal
Protein	11.0 g
Carboydrate	72.0 g
of which sugars	2.0 g
Fat	1.0 g
of which saturates	0.2 g
Fibre	3.0 g
Sodium	trace
This pack contains 2 servings.	

A label on a packet of biscuits gives information per 100 g and per biscuit which is even more useful.

Average values	per biscuit	per 100 g
Energy	165 kJ/39 kcal	1760 kJ/420 kcal
Protein	0.4	4.5
Carboydrate	8.2	87.0
of which sugar	5.4	57.7
Fat	0.5	5.5
of which saturated	0.2	2.3
Fibre	0.1	1.1
Sodium	trace	0.3

Ingredients on labels

The list of ingredients on a label can give an idea of what is in a food but it is not as helpful as the nutritional label. Often harmless ingredients can sound very unnatural and vice versa.

The most important thing about ingredients is that they are listed in order of quantity, with the ingredient of which there is most in the product listed first. So for example, if 'sugar' is listed first in the ingredients list there is more sugar in that product than anything else!

Double check by looking at the nutritional label as the ingredients list alone does not give the full picture.

Fat, sugar and salt		
	A lot is more than	A little is less than
Fat	17.5 g per 100 g	3.0 g per 100 g
Saturated fat	5.0 g per 100 g	1.5 g per 100 g
Sugar	22.5 g per 100 g	5.0 g per 100 g
Salt	1.5 g per 100 g (or 0.6 g sodium)	0.3 g per 100 g (or 0.1 g sodium)

How to decide which food to buy

Fat, sugar and salt are the three main nutrients that most health professionals are concerned about in food.

First, check the nutritional label to see how much fat, sugar and salt is contained in the product. These are the most important nutrients on the label to check. Some foods contain a lot of fat, sugar and salt and you need to be aware of that when making your choice of what to buy. The table above shows what counts as a lot and what counts as a little when it comes to fat, sugar and salt.

- Then check roughly what a serving size is. If this information is not given check the number of grams in the packet—this will be written somewhere on the front or back of the packet. Then work out roughly how much of the food your child will be eating. For example, if a packet contains 10 biscuits and 250 g is written on the outside of the packet, then each biscuit weighs about 25 g. This means the values given per 100 g account for about 4 biscuits.

- Next, check the ingredients. Although the ingredients list is not as helpful as the nutritional list it will tell you which ingredients predominate in the product as they are listed in order of quantity. So if sugar, for example, is listed second you know that the product contains a great deal of sugar.

- Lastly, compare the brand you buy with other brands. Is there another brand that is lower in sugar, fat or salt? If you are buying a processed-type product, does a less processed version provide less sugar, for example, or the same amount? Only by comparing with other brands, can you get a real feel for what you are buying.

Certain foods are naturally high in sugar, fat and salt but this does not mean that they are unhealthy foods. For example, cheddar cheese is high in fat and salt but it is good for your child because it is high in protein and calcium.

If you compare brands of cheddar cheese you will find that they all contain roughly the same amounts of fat and salt. So you should include cheese in your child's diet but not too much of it. One or two portions a day, depending on your child's overall diet, should be fine.

Fat

Many important parts of the body rely on fat to function properly so fat is not always bad, especially when children are concerned. Children need more fat in their diets than adults with fat providing 35 per cent of their daily energy as compared with 30 per cent for adults. However, the 2005 National Children's Food Survey showed that almost half of Irish children aged between 5 and 12 years receive more than 35 per cent of their daily energy from fat; this is too high a proportion. Too much fat in the diet can cause overweight and obesity in addition to raised blood cholesterol and other health problems.

What's really important, however, is the type of fat consumed.

Polyunsaturated fat, from, for example, vegetable oil, sunflower oil and oily fish, is very good for your child's health and wellbeing.

Monounsaturated fat from, for example, olive oil and avocados, is also very beneficial to your child.

Saturated fat, however, from foods like fatty and processed meat, ready-meals, biscuits, cakes and confectionery, is not good for your child's health. An excess of saturated fat in the diet can increase cholesterol levels, particularly LDL or 'bad' cholesterol.

Trans fat is worse again. It is found mainly in processed foods such as ready-meals, biscuits, cakes, crackers and confectionery. Trans fat is a specific type of fat formed when liquid oils are made into solid fats, part of a manufacturing process called 'hydrogenation'. Many fast-food companies use this hydrogenated vegetable oil to cook their food, making the food high in trans fat also. 'Shortening', often used in baking, contains trans fat and this means that many baked goods contain trans fat.

Trans fat not only increases 'bad' cholesterol, it also decreases 'good' cholesterol. This two-tiered assault makes trans fat even more dangerous than saturated fats.

While the effects of trans fat are obviously of great concern, people are generally eating far more saturated fat in their diets than trans fat so that at present saturated fat is more of a health issue than trans fat.

Dairy products like milk, yogurt and cheese also contain saturated fat. However, in all other ways they are a very healthy food group. This is where you have to weigh up the pros and cons of a food and use your common sense. Yes, there is saturated fat in whole milk but it also contains protein, calcium and vitamins. Compare this with the saturated fat in a biscuit which gives your child really no other nutritional benefits.

too much fat will cause your child to become overweight
Remember, too much fat, whether saturated, polyunsaturated monounsaturated, or trans fat, will cause your child to gain excess weight.

how to decide if a food is healthy
- Check the nutritional label to see how high it is in fat, sugar and salt.
- Work out how much fat, sugar and salt is contained in each portion
- Check the ingredients.
- Compare the food to other brands.

So, when looking at a food label, look at the fat content of the food as, whether your child is overweight or not, it is good to be aware of how much fat is in different foods. Above all, check the content of saturated fat as it is not good for health and should be kept to a minimum. (The only exception to this is when a child is failing to gain weight and is undernourished. In this case we recommend any type of fat to help with weight gain until a healthy weight is achieved. See Chapter 11.)

At present, it is not compulsory to list trans fat on the nutritional label so it can be difficult to know how much trans fat is in a food. If 'partially hydrogenated vegetable oil' or 'hydrogenated vegetable oil' or 'hydrogenates' appears in the ingredients list, the food is likely to contain trans fat. The higher in the ingredients list the trans fat appears the more of it there is in the food. You and your child should eat as little trans fat as possible.

> **a little butter does no harm**
>
> There is nothing wrong with giving your child butter if you make sure not to overdo it. While butter is high in saturated fat, small amounts will do no harm.

Since butter is natural and margarine contains additives and possibly trans fat should I stick to butter?

Butter is made from animal fat and margarine is made from vegetable fat. Butter contains about 80 g fat in total per 100 g and soft margarines contain less (approximately 60 g per 100 g). Low-fat margarines contain even less total fat. However, butter is very high in saturated fat (54 g per 100 g). Soft margarine contains far less saturated fat (approximately 7–15 g per 100 g). Margarine is also often fortified with vitamin D and other vitamins.

Even though soft margarine may contain some trans fat, the extra amounts of saturated fat in butter makes soft margarine a better choice in terms of heart health. The Irish Heart Foundation and the American Heart Association recommend the use of soft margarine as a substitute for butter.

> **tips to cut down on your child's intake of added sugar**
>
> ▪ Don't allow soft drinks except on special occasions.
> ▪ Don't give sugary treats except on occasion (not every day). Give fruit instead.
> ▪ Encourage milk and water as a drink.
> ▪ If giving juice, look for one with 'no added sugar'.
> ▪ Avoid giving a sugary cereal in the morning.
> ▪ Compare brands of yogurt and pick one with the smallest amount of sugar.

Sugar

Sugar to most people means the type of sugar we put in our tea or coffee or that is used in baking. However, there are many different types of sugars present in a whole range of foods. The sugar in breast milk and cow's milk is called 'lactose'. Sugars such as fructose are also naturally present in fruits and vegetables.

Generally, naturally present sugars are not bad for your child's teeth or health. It is 'added sugars' which are extracted from certain foods and added to other foods that are especially bad for your child's teeth. These include sucrose (table sugar), maltose, glucose, dextrose, invert sugar and fructose.

Eating too much sugar as a child leads to tooth decay and obesity. It may also displace more important nutrients from the diet, for example calcium and iron. The National Children's Food Survey (IUNA 2005) showed that Irish children aged 5–12 years are taking almost 2 glasses of sugary drink per day in addition to other sugary treats. This is far too much sugar.

Check the label

Sugar, unlike fat, does not offer any great nutritional benefits apart from giving your child calories for energy, so you should choose foods that are low in added sugar, where possible. Check the label and compare it to the 'a lot' and 'a little' values above.

Check the ingredients also; if sugar is one of the first ingredients listed, there is a lot of added sugar in that food. Breakfast cereals and yogurts can be quite high in sugar so it is a good idea to compare brands and pick the lower sugar options where possible.

You could always give your child a little natural yogurt and sweeten it with a fruit purée instead of sugar. However, if your child is not eating a lot of sugary cereals, biscuits, confectionary and drinks, sugar intake is probably at a reasonably low level.

diabetes
Eating too much sugar does not directly cause diabetes but it could cause someone to become overweight and being overweight might cause them to develop Type II diabetes (Type I diabetes is not caused by being over-weight). There is no conclusive scientific evidence to date that shows that eating too much sugar causes hyperactivity.

Salt

Diets high in salt have been associated with high blood pressure which in turn increases the risk of cardiovascular disease. Children also have immature kidneys which aren't able to cope with large amounts of salt in their diet. Furthermore, giving children a taste for salt will more than likely cause them to take more salt during adulthood and increase their risk of high blood pressure and cardiovascular disease.

While most people try to reduce the salt added at the table or in cooking, it is the salt already in certain foods that is contributing most to our diets. About 70 per cent of the salt we eat everyday comes from processed foods alone.

Many groups such as the UK Foods Standards Agency have been targeting food manufacturers, asking them to reduce the amount of salt in their products.

Food Safety Authority of Ireland (FSAI) recommendations on salt intake	
Age	Maximum daily intake
7–12 months	1 g
1–3 years	2 g
4–6 years	3 g

salt and sodium

Sometimes 'sodium' is written instead of salt. To find the salt content multiply the sodium number by 2.5. For example, if a food has 0.5 g sodium per 100 g multiply 0.5 by 2.5 which gives 1.25. Therefore this food has 1.25 g salt per 100 g.

foods particularly high in salt

- Meat products (e.g. sausages, frankfurters, rashers, cured meats)
- Packaged soups
- Ready-meals, pizzas etc.
- Pre-packaged sauces
- Stock cubes

Salt content of different foods*

Food	Salt content
1 regular sized sausage, grilled	0.5 g
1 cocktail sized sausage	0.25
1 sausage roll	0.75 g
1 rasher (lean) 25g	1.2 g
1 large slice ham (30 g, from packet)	0.70g
2 fish fingers	0.3–0.5 g
¼ of a 9 inch pizza	0.6 g
1 portion cheese dip with sticks (50g)	0.75 g
1 individual portion children's cheese (20g)	0.50
Unprocessed cheddar cheese (28g)	0.5 g
1 soup in a cup	2.25 g
1 slice white bread 30g	0.4 g
1 slice whole meal bread	0.4 g
1 potato waffle	0.5 g
2 Weetabix	0.2 g
1 bowl Ready Brek (30g)	< 0.25 g
1 bowl corn flakes (30g)	0.5 g
1 bowl shredded wheat (30g)	trace
1 bowl Shreddies (30g)	0.2 g
1 bowl bran flakes (30g)	0.4 g

*amounts vary from brand to brand

Is there a danger of eating too little salt?

With salt added to so many foods it would be very difficult to eat none at all, however hard you try. Some children with certain medical conditions may have a higher need for salt in their diets but the average healthy child does not.

Check the label for salt content and see if it constitutes 'a little' or 'a lot' according to the values on page 136. Bear in mind also how much salt the FSAI recommends for your child. A product containing 0.3 g salt per 100 g is considered low in salt but 100 g of that product will provide a 7–12-month-old baby with almost a third of the maximum recommended intake of salt per day. Visit www.salt.gov.uk for more tips on avoiding salt.

Food additives

Food additives are substances added to foods to perform certain technological functions such as colouring, sweetening or preserving the food. They can be natural or manufactured. Each additive falls into one of the following categories: acidity regulators, antioxidants, colours, emulsifiers, flavour enhancers, flavourings, gelling agents, preservatives, stabilisers, raising agents, thickeners, and sweeteners.

In the EU, food additives are evaluated for safety by the EU Scientific Committee on Food, an expert advisory panel. Only additives that have been authorised by this body may be included in foods sold in the EU—this applies to all the member states. Where a food contains an additive this must be stated on the label by category (for example, preservative or colouring) with *either* the full name *or* the E number. There are very strict guidelines and laws to which manufacturers must conform when using food additives.

Categories and roles of food additives

Category	Role	Examples
Acidity regulators	Change or maintain the acidity or alkalinity of a food.	Tartaric acid or E334
Antioxidants	Added to foods to prevent them from 'going off' when in contact with air.	Vitamin C (ascorbic acid) or E300
Colours	Added to foods to make them look more attractive.	Caramel or E150a
Emulsifiers	Allow oil- and water-based ingredients to be mixed together equally and prevent them separating.	Lecithins or E322
Flavour enhancers	Bring out flavour in a food without adding a flavour of their own.	Monosodium glutamate or MSG or E621
Gelling agents and thickeners	Modify texture and provide stability.	Sodium alginates or E401
Preservatives	Prolong the shelf-life of foods by preventing them from being destroyed by bacteria and fungi.	Sulphur Dioxide or E220
Raising agents	Liberate gas and thereby increase volume of dough or batter.	Sodium bicarbonate (E500)
Stabilisers	Give food good texture and mouth-feel.	Sucroglycerides or E474
Sweeteners	Used instead of sugar as they are lower in calories.	Sorbitol or E420

The Food Safety Authority of Ireland looked at different food types and the percentage of brands within each type of food product that contained food additives. They found that food additives were contained in *all* brands of diet soft drinks, low-fat spreads and pâté and in almost all brands of regular soft drinks, sausages, bacon and ham, chocolate confectionery, desserts and sugar confectionery.

Children and food additives

Regulations do not permit sweeteners and colours to be added to foods aimed at infants (less than 1 year old) and young children (3 years old and under) with some exceptions.

Specific legislation regulates the additives in foods such as infant formula, follow-on formula and weaning foods. Rules relating to food additives in children's foods are all EU directives so the same rules apply throughout the EU.

Which food additives should I be trying to avoid?

All food additives have been tested and considered safe so they are all suitable for human consumption. Many additives are necessary for a number of reasons, one of the main ones being to prolong shelf life.

If you wish to avoid food additives, the best way is to buy as few pre-manufactured foods as possible. Read labels to see what food additives are in the foods you are buying.

It is healthier to eat as few processed foods as possible as they tend to be higher in fat, sugar and salt. So if you follow healthy eating guidelines and provide your child with lots of fresh fruit, vegetables, meat and fish, you will not be giving too many food additives anyway.

Remember, however, that manufacturers don't have to label food additives as E numbers but instead may list them under their full name, for example 'ascorbic acid' instead of 'E300'. So although no E numbers may appear in the ingredients list this doesn't mean there aren't any food additives in the product.

Do food additives cause hyperactivity in children?

In the late 1970s Dr Ben F. Feingold produced a theory that food additives caused hyperactivity in children. From this came the 'Feingold diet' which was free of all the substances he deemed to cause hyperactivity in children. The theory was investigated by other researchers but until recently there was no conclusive evidence backing Dr Feingold's theory. However, in 2007, research on the effects of food additives, carried out by Southampton University, was published. The study examined the effects of different mixes of food colourings combined with the preservative sodium benzoate on the activity of one group of children aged 3 years and on another group aged 8–9 years. The study found a link between the colours used in the research and the increased levels of hyperactivity in the children. The colours used were Sunset yellow (E110), Quinoline yellow (E104), Carmoisine (E122), Allura red (E129), Tartrazine (E102) and Ponceau 4R (E124).

It is not clear from the study whether it was an individual colour or a combination of colourings that caused the hyperactivity. No individual colour has been identified as a cause of hyperactivity. It is most unlikely that in normal circumstances a child would eat a food or foods combining all the colours listed above. However, following this study, the UK Food Standards Agency now recommends that if a

'additive free' claims

Beware of claims made about foods being free of food additives. Remember, sugar is not considered a food additive — just because a food says 'no added sweeteners or colours' does not mean it is not full of sugar!

child shows signs of hyperactivity or ADHD (Attention Deficit Hyperactivity Disorder) it may be useful to try to eliminate the colours used in the Southampton study from his or her diet.

Genetically modified (GM) foods

Animals and plants are made up of millions of cells. These cells contain genes which are made up of DNA. Genes are passed on from generation to generation and affect everything from the colour of eyes in humans to the colour of flowers in plants.

Scientists can identify certain genes in plants and their role within the plant. Technology is available to change or modify genes in order, for example, to increase the amount of vitamins in a tomato, or to make a plant more resistant to infection. This is done by transferring genes from other organisms that are resistant to the infection into the plant in question.

Genetically modified (GM) food contains, or is produced from, genetically modified organisms. Most GM foods are made from GM plants, especially maize and soya bean. A GM food may contain one or a number of GM ingredients.

GM foods offer great potential benefits. For example, wheat with increased levels of folic acid could help prevent spina bifida in infants or crops could be designed to survive in harsher climates in developing countries.

However, a number of concerns have been raised about GM foods. Some of these relate to food safety, transfer of antibiotic resistance to humans, environmental concerns about disrupting eco-systems and moral and ethical concerns.

At present there are only a small number of GM foods available on the Irish market compared to the US and Canada where there is a much larger range available. Ingredients from genetically modified maize, soya bean, rapeseed oil, sugar beet and cotton are allowed to be sold in Ireland.

Soya beans are used extensively in processed foods. Soya lecithin, a food additive (E322), very frequently seen in the ingredients of foods, may or may not be from a GM source. Breads, biscuits, infant formula, confectionery, cereals and chocolate products may contain GM soya ingredients.

GM maize is also often found in foods such as beer, margarine, salad dressing, taco shells, tortilla chips and bakery products.

GM food legislation

GM foods are subjected to an extensive range of safety tests before being allowed to be sold here. The Food Safety Authority of Ireland evaluates each GM food separately to ensure that it meets strict criteria for safety. It carries out frequent surveys to monitor the use and labelling of GM ingredients in Ireland.

A survey carried out in 2007 found no breaches of GM food legislation. The study took a total of 97 foods and tested samples of each for GM ingredients. GM soya bean was found in 13 of the 97 products but not at a level of more than 0.9 per cent, the permitted level.

Labelling GM foods

At present in Ireland, if more than 0.9 per cent of a food or ingredient is from a GM source, it must be labelled accordingly. A food labelled 'GM free' must not contain any GM ingredients at all. Any food labeled as 'organic' must also be free from GM ingredients.

A leaflet on GM foods produced by the the Food Safety Authority of Ireland can be downloaded from www.fsai.ie or call 1890 336677 for a free copy.

Organic foods

Organic food is usually taken to mean a food that has been produced without artificial fertilisers and has not been subject to treatment with synthetic pesticides or growth promoters of any type, including hormones and antibiotics. Organic food is more expensive than its regular equivalent, as a less intensive style of farming is involved. Official certification bodies inspect all farms producing organic produce.

In Ireland, fruit and vegetables comprise the largest organic food type; meats, dairy and other organic products make up the balance. Larger supermarkets usually have separate organic food areas. Local farmers' markets held throughout the country, usually at weekends, offer fresh organic foods direct from the producer.

Is organic food superior?

It is still a matter of public and scientific debate whether organic food is superior with respect to nutritional content or quality.

Organic fruit and vegetables can be expected to contain fewer agrochemical residues than the conventional alternative. However, there are strict limits as to the amount of agrochemical residues allowed in conventional foods, and in practice most conventional food contains less than the maximum allowed. Both types of foods are likely to contain some environmental contaminants.

Organic farmers claim that their method is less harmful to the environment and to food producers, and they place strong emphasis on animal welfare.

Ultimately, the choice is yours. Whatever the origin of the food you buy, strive for a well-balanced diet using fresh produce.

Children's foods

In the last number of years there has been a huge increase in the number of foods on the market aimed specifically at children. 'Children's foods' sections have appeared in the supermarket, with products ranging from yogurts and breakfast cereals to bite-sized breaded chicken and mini pizzas.

The first thing to say about this trend is that there is no need for special foods for children. Often adults have an idea that children can only be given mini-yogurts or children's breakfast cereals but this is not the case. Children can be given almost any adult cereal—with the exception of cereals containing whole or chopped nuts. This whole concept of children needing special foods was created by marketing experts in food companies around the world.

Most of the time, 'children's foods' are higher in sugar than their 'adult' counterparts, obviously to appeal to children's preference for sweeter tastes. Children's foods can also be higher in fat and salt. Not all children's foods are bad but it is important to check the labels and look at the sugar, fat and salt content so that you know what is in the product you are buying. It can be quite interesting, too, to compare it to an adult equivalent.

Children's yogurts and fromage frais

There is now a huge range of children's yogurts on the market. Many of them are fromage frais rather than plain yogurt. Fromage frais, which is originally from Belgium and northern France, is actually a cheese, as the name suggests, not a yogurt. It is made like a cheese except that the curds are not allowed to solidify and instead take on a consistency more like yogurt. Generally, cream is added to improve the flavour. Fromage frais is neither more nor less healthy than yogurt—it depends on how much sugar and fat are added.

Before you buy a yogurt or fromage frais for your child, look at the nutritional labels of each one and compare them. Pick one that is comparatively lower in sugar and fat. Most children's yogurts or fromage frais contain more than 8 g of sugar per 100 g. Some of this sugar is lactose which is naturally present in milk and is not harmful to a child's teeth. There is about 4.5 g per 100 g of lactose in yogurt and 3 g per 100 g in fromage frais. So, whatever the total amount of sugar in the product, 3–4.5 g of this is lactose, depending on whether it is fromage frais or yogurt.

include cheese in your child's diet
Cheese, being high in fat and salt, may appear to be a very unhealthy food. However, it is an excellent source of protein, containing about 25 g per 100 g or 7 g per portion (the same as a slice of meat). It is also very high in calcium, containing about 700 mg per 100 g, or 200 mg per 28 g portion, almost as much as a glass of milk and a quarter of a child's Recommended Daily Allowance. So you should definitely include cheese in your child's diet but restrict it to 1 or 2 portions a day depending on age.

Portion sizes of children's yogurts and fromage frais vary from 60 g to 100 g so remember also to keep in mind the portion size when reading the label. Beware of claims on the label such as 'a source of calcium' as this may distract attention away from the fact that the yogurt is full of sugar or fat. Read the label and decide for yourself. Dessert-type yogurts should be treated in the same way as any other treat food, such as chocolate or ice-cream, and given occasionally only.

Unless your child is overweight it is fine to give full-fat yogurt or fromage frais. Don't give a child younger than 5 years diet yogurt or fromage frais as the added sweeteners could cause stomach upsets. If you want to avoid the sugar in most yogurts and fromage frais, you could give your child natural yogurt (only 4.5 g sugar per 100 g—all lactose) and sweeten it with some puréed or chopped fruit.

Children's cheeses

A number of cheeses are now available specifically for children. Most are a version of cheddar cheese, processed to make it 'spreadable' or 'bendable' in some way. Cheese products are all over the 20 g per 100 g fat mark that we consider 'high fat'. This is because cheese itself is high in fat. Regular unprocessed cheddar cheese contains about 30 g fat, 20 g of which is saturated fat. So processed cheese is no worse than unprocessed in this regard.

Cheese is also high in salt. Unprocessed cheese contains about 1.75 g salt (0.7 g sodium) per 100 g which again falls into our category of 'a lot' of salt. A portion size of cheese is about the size of a matchbox (28 g) and this contains about 0.5 g salt.

Processed cheeses tend to contain more salt, some as much as 3.25 g (1.4 g sodium) per 100 g. So look out for brands which contain less salt and go for those ones. Remember, to find out how much salt there is, multiply the value for sodium by 2.5.

Products consisting of cheese as a 'dip' with breadsticks and cheese with crackers in individual portions can be significantly higher in fat and salt. Again some may not be too high so be sure to compare brands.

Most of the figures above relate to cheddar cheese as it is the cheese most eaten in Ireland. Some other cheeses, such as mozzarella and feta, are slightly lower in fat than cheddar but they also contain less calcium and protein.

the very best breakfast cereals contain

- Less than 0.3 g salt per 100 g
- Less than 5 g sugar per 100 g
- Less than 3 g fat per 100 g
- More than 6 g fibre per 100 g

Children's breakfast cereals

There has been a lot of controversy about children's breakfast cereals with a number of consumer groups declaring that they are unhealthy for children. The majority of children's breakfast cereals certainly are higher in sugar than 'adult' cereals. They may or may not be higher in fat and salt. There is absolutely no need, however, to give your child a children's cereal. Children can eat any cereal on the shelf except for muesli, which may contain whole or chopped nuts. Remember an 'average' bowl of cereal for a child between the ages of 1 and 5 years is 10–30 g (1–3 tablespoons).

Sugar in cereals When choosing a breakfast cereal, it's best to pick one that contains less than 5 g sugar per 100 g. Not many cereals meet these criteria but those that do include Weetabix, Ready Brek, Oatibix, Shredded Wheat and, of course, porridge which is always a good choice as it is also high in soluble fibre. Don't forget to check supermarket own brands also to see if they are within the recommended range.

Some children's breakfast cereals contain as much as 37 g sugar per 100 g. One bowl of such a cereal provides 11 g sugar which is almost 3 teaspoons of sugar. Even if you managed to give your child a breakfast cereal containing less than 10 g sugar per 100 g you would be doing well. Every level teaspoon of sugar put on a child's cereal is adding 4 g of sugar.

Fibre in cereals Cereals are a great way to provide fibre to your child so pick one that has more than 6 g of fibre per 100 g. Fibre not only helps to keep your child's bowel healthy but it also keeps him or her fuller for longer. Porridge is an excellent source of soluble fibre.

Salt in cereals It is strange to think of salt being in cereal but some cereals can be quite high in salt. It can be very hard to find a cereal that fits into the category of 'a little' salt, i.e. less than 0.3 g per 100 g.

Some cereals contain as much as 1.75 g salt (0.7 g sodium) per 100 g which translates as 0.5 g salt per bowl. This is quite a lot of salt for a cereal and when your child may be only allowed 3 g salt per day, this is a significant contribution to that amount.

Compare labels and be aware of how much salt is in the different brands of cereal.

Fat in cereals Breakfast cereals by nature are generally low in fat as they are mainly a carbohydrate-based food. It is best to pick a cereal that has less than 3 g fat per 100 g. Quite a number of cereals on the market fall into this category.

Added vitamins and minerals in cereals One of the biggest selling points of breakfast cereals is their added vitamins and minerals. If your child's diet is restricted in any way due to allergies or 'fussiness', giving cereals can be a useful way of obtaining the necessary vitamins or minerals.

Different breakfast cereals are fortified with different amounts and types of vitamins and minerals. The majority have added B vitamins and folic acid and some also contain added vitamin D, vitamin C, iron and calcium. The added vitamins and minerals are listed on the packet along with the other nutritional information. Some breakfast cereals can provide up to half of your child's daily requirement for iron.

It sounds like most breakfast cereals are full of sugar and salt, should I avoid giving them to my child completely?

The answer to this is no. A breakfast cereal that is low in sugar, fat and salt and high in fibre is a very healthy option in the morning, especially with the added milk. You will need to check the nutritional labels to find one of the handful of cereals that is a fairly good fit for all these criteria. If you then find that your child doesn't like this cereal, you could always make a deal that it is eaten from Monday to Friday and the cereal that he or she prefers on Saturday and/or Sunday. You could also put a handful of high-fibre cereal into a bowl of the preferred cereal.

It is better that your child eat a sugary cereal for breakfast than no food at all, if that is the choice.

Common nutritional problems in toddlers

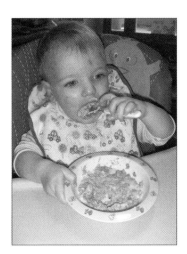

Just as babies can have problems related to feeding, toddlers also can have difficulties in this area. Constipation and diarrhoea are quite common in toddlers and are often related to diet.

Toddlers also tend to pick up more infections than babies; those who were breastfed no longer have the immunological protection of breast milk and toddlers tend to mix more with one another, passing on infection in daycare or play groups. Sometimes after a number of infections in a row a child may not gain enough weight which can be worrying for a parent.

In this chapter we cover a number of common nutritional problems we see in toddlers and advise on how to cope with them if they arise and how to avoid them happening in the first place.

Iron-deficiency anaemia

Anaemia is a condition in which the red blood cells, which carry oxygen around the body, are deficient in quality. Iron-deficiency anaemia occurs when there is insufficient iron in the diet. Because they are growing so rapidly, infants and toddlers have a high requirement for iron and if they don't get enough in their diet may become anaemic. Children with anaemia often lose their appetites and become tired, listless and irritable; their immunity may also be compromised so that they pick up infections more easily. There is increasing evidence that iron-deficiency anaemia can affect a child's brain development.

Alarmingly, a study carried out on children in Ireland found that almost 10 per cent of toddlers had iron-deficiency anaemia. The study showed that children who had been given cow's milk as a main drink before the age of 1 year were at the highest risk of developing the condition.

How to prevent your child from developing iron deficiency anaemia

- Don't give cow's milk as a main drink until the age of 1 year.
- Don't let your child (1 year old or older) drink more than 600–700 ml of cow's milk a day.
- Do introduce iron-rich foods—red meat, eggs, beans and lentils—from the age of 6 months.
- Don't let your child drink tea as this can affect the absorption of iron from food.

daily iron requirements
Children aged 1–3 years need 8 mg of iron every day; children aged 4–6 years need 9 mg iron daily.

The following foods are rich in iron:

- Red meat—beef, lamb, mutton, pork, bacon
- Oily fish
- Eggs
- Beans and lentils (baked beans are fine)
- Dark green vegetables
- Dried fruit
- Wholemeal bread
- Fortified breakfast cereals

Iron content of certain foods

Food	Portion size	Iron (mg)
Minced beef	2 tablespoons	1.5
Chicken breast	½ small (50 g)	0.2
Lean rasher	1	0.2
Sausage	1	0.2
Egg	1	1.0
Salmon	½ average steak (50 g)	0.25
Sardines	1 tinned sardine	0.6
Tuna	½ tin (50 g)	0.8
White fish	½ small fillet (50 g)	0.2
Special K	medium bowl (30 g)	3.0
Weetabix	2 biscuits	5.0
Ready Brek	medium bowl (30 g)	3.5
Cheerios	medium bowl (30 g)	3.5
Wholemeal bread	1 slice (35 g)	1.0
Baked beans	200g (1 small tin)	3.0
Baked beans	1 tablespoon	0.6
Tofu, firm	90 g	3.0
Kidney beans, cooked	3 heaped tablespoons (105 g)	2.6
Lentils, cooked	3 tablespoons	4.2
1 portion cooked spinach	2 tablespoons (80 g)	1.3
Raisins	1 tablespoon	1.0
Lamb, roast	1 slice, 30 g	0.5

As you can see, when it comes to meat and fish, red meat and oily fish contain the most iron.

How do I find out if my child is iron deficient?

A simple blood test—a full blood count—carried out by your GP will show if your child is anaemic or not. Your GP may also check the level of ferritin in the blood to assess your child's iron stores.

People may tell you to see if your child is pale under the eyes or pale in the face but really the only way to know for sure if your child is anaemic is to get a full blood count done. Iron-deficiency anaemia is serious but also very treatable.

If your child is iron deficient your GP will prescribe an iron supplement for a few weeks or months. This should cure the anaemia over a number of weeks. Iron supplements can cause constipation and may make your child's stools become darker.

If your child is having problems taking the supplement, ask your GP or pharmacist for advice. Don't stop giving your child a prescribed iron supplement for iron-deficiency anaemia unless advised to do so by your GP or pharmacist.

iron in meat

The iron from meat sources is absorbed up to 7 times more easily than the iron in cereals, vegetables and fruits. Try to give your toddler iron from meat sources regularly — aim to give red meat at least 3 times a week.

fruit and vegetables high in vitamin C

Oranges, kiwis, lemons, berries, peppers, broccoli, tomatoes, unsweetened fruit juice

Three easy ways to boost your toddler's iron intake
- Give red meat three times a week.
- Provide other good sources of iron like oily fish, baked beans and eggs.
- Choose a breakfast cereal with added iron and give it to your child with a small glass of unsweetened juice to help absorb the iron.

Vitamin C and iron absorption
Vitamin C helps the body absorb iron from non-meat foods (vegetables, cereals, eggs, fruits) so it is good to take a drink or food containing vitamin C with these foods. For example, a small glass of unsweetened orange juice in the morning helps the body to absorb iron from iron-fortified cereal.

The girl who wanted to eat dog biscuits

In our clinics we often see children with iron-deficiency anaemia but there are a few cases that really stand out. One such was an 18-month-old girl, Aisling, who came into A&E with decreased appetite and energy. The doctors did a full blood count and saw that Aisling had severe iron-deficiency anaemia. Her parents said that she was drinking over 2 litres of milk a day and didn't seem interested in eating solids at all.

Iron-deficiency anaemia is often seen in children who drink too much milk and eat very little solid food. This is because milk contains no iron. Aisling was so full drinking milk, she had no appetite for eating solid food such as meat, eggs and vegetables which would have provided her with iron. Iron-deficiency anaemia itself causes poor appetite so, as Aisling's appetite got worse, she ate even less.

The doctors put Aisling on an iron supplement and within weeks her mother reported that she was a 'different child'. Within 6 months Aisling's iron level was back to normal.

One interesting thing about Aisling is that her mother reported that she wanted to eat dog biscuits all the time when she was anaemic. This behaviour of eating things that aren't human food is called 'pica' and is frequently seen in children with iron-deficiency anaemia. Over the years we have heard stories of iron-deficient children eating various different things from plaster to earth. Pica can also be caused by other medical conditions.

Diarrhoea

Amost all toddlers get diarrhoea at one stage or another. Diarrhoea is defined as passing frequent, loose, watery stools. It may only last for a day or two or linger on for a week or longer. Generally diarrhoea is caused by a 'bug' or infection (usually viral).

If your child has diarrhoea it is important to keep him or her well-hydrated. One of the best ways to do this is to get an oral rehydration solution such as Dioralyte or Rapolyte from the pharmacist and give it as directed. Oral rehydration solutions come as a sachet of powder that you make up with water and they provide not only fluid but also salts that can be lost during periods of vomiting or diarrhoea. If your child won't drink the solution try another flavour – they usually come in a range of flavours. Try to give your child a cup of Dioralyte or Rapolyte every time a loose stool is passed, in addition to the normal fluid intake.

Remember, young children become dehydrated very easily and this can be very dangerous. If you are in any way concerned, bring your child to the GP or hospital A&E.

Should I give fluids only, and no solid food, when my child has diarrhoea?

Traditionally when an adult or child had diarrhoea, it was advised that they take fluids only and avoid solid food for a day or two. However, nowadays early re-introduction of solid food during an episode of diarrhoea is recommended. Oral re-hydration solutions should be given for 3–4 hours followed by re-introduction of normal feeding thereafter.

However, if your child seems to get worse after feeding, don't give milk and solids for 24 hours and give the rehydration solution during this time.

Toddler diarrhoea

Toddler diarrhoea is the name given to a type of unexplained diarrhoea in children aged from 1 to 6 years. The diarrhoea is 'chronic' which means it has been happening for a period of weeks or months. The child is healthy with plenty of energy, gaining weight well and has no other symptoms except watery, frequent, stools with often identifiable pieces of food in them.

cut out the juice

If your child is having constant diarrhoea it is very important to cut out juice from the diet completely or limit it to half a glass a day.

The three Fs: fat, fruit juice and fluid

Making some key dietary changes may help clear up toddler diarrhoea. We have named this approach 'the 3 Fs'—fat, fruit juice, fluid—and have found it to be effective in treating this type of diarrhoea.

Fat An infant's diet of breast milk or infant formula is high in fat (50 per cent energy from fat). However, when children are weaned onto solids, the fat content of their diet reduces greatly, especially if they are poor milk-drinkers after the age of 1 year. Fat is one thing that slows down the movement of food through the gut. Therefore when fat is reduced in a child's diet, food can move more quickly through the gut and often comes out watery and looks only partially digested.

In order to increase the fat in your child's diet, aim to provide 600 ml full-fat milk a day, taken as 3 glasses of 200 ml, spread out over breakfast, lunch and dinner or between meals. Full-fat yogurt and cheese also provide fat, in a more nutritious way. You could also add some olive oil in cooking and put sunflower spread or similar on bread and in sandwiches. For example, plain pasta with a tomato-based sauce is a very low-fat meal. You could make it higher in fat by adding a handful of parmesan cheese to the sauce or by drizzling a little olive oil on the pasta before adding the sauce. If your child won't eat this, give a glass of full-fat milk to drink with the pasta and tomato sauce and a full-fat yogurt for dessert.

Don't try to increase fat in your child's diet by giving junk foods.

Fruit juice Toddlers usually love fruit juice. However, not only does drinking a lot of juice displace other foods from the diet that might contain fat, but the juice itself has been implicated as one of the major contributing factors to toddler diarrhoea. One of the reasons for this may be that juice, especially apple juice, is high in a sugar called fructose which may be hard for some children to absorb. Some juices also contain sorbitol (another type of sugar) which can also contribute to the problem. A lot of cases of toddler diarrhoea are completely cured by simply cutting out juice.

Fluid Drinking large amounts of fluid is another cause of toddler diarrhoea. This is mainly because children who drink a lot of fluid tend to eat less solid food and therefore tend to eat less fat which can help prevent toddler diarrhoea. In addition to this, as we have seen, if the fluid is juice the sugars in the juice itself will probably make the problem even worse.

Ideally, a child between the ages of 1 and 5 should be drinking at the very most 1200–1500 ml of fluid a day, depending on age (1-year-olds taking 1200 ml and 5-year-olds taking 1500 ml) *and this includes milk.* Unless there is a medical reason why your child needs to drink a lot of fluid, this will be more than enough to keep your child hydrated. Any more fluid than this will start affecting the intake of solids.

> **lactose intolerance**
> is not an allergy. It occasionally occurs after an episode of diarrhoea and is usually temporary.

If the diarrhoea does not clear up after you've made the above dietary changes, bring your child to your GP for further investigation. If your child is overweight you may need to see a dietitian before increasing the fat in the diet.

Lactose intolerance

Occasionally, following a dose of diarrhoea, a child develops temporary lactose intolerance which causes prolonged diarrhoea after the infection has cleared up. (Lactose is the naturally occurring sugar in milk.) Lactose intolerance can also be an inherited condition but it is rare in Caucasian children. Treatment is the same regardless of the cause.

If your child has had a bug that caused diarrhoea and does not show any signs of improvement after a week, a temporary lactose intolerance may have developed. In this case you need to avoid giving cow's milk and provide an alternative such as soya milk with added calcium for about 4–6 weeks. By this time, the gut will have healed and your child will be able to drink cow's milk again. Hard cheeses contain only small amounts of lactose so your child might be able to tolerate them. Yogurt also contains lactose but the fermentation of the yogurt during manufacturing destroys most of it so your child may be able to tolerate it. However, if your child gets diarrhoea again after taking cheese or yogurt, avoid it during the 4–6 week period.

The lactose intolerance may clear up in a shorter period than 4–6 weeks. You can try with cow's milk before this and if it is tolerated without any diarrhoea, then the lactose intolerance has cleared up.

Lactose intolerance is often dose-dependent. This means that your child may be able to tolerate small amounts of lactose in foods. Lactose is found in a whole range of foods such as biscuits, sausages, baby jars, cereals and many other products. You should read food labels to check whether foods contain lactose or not.

If you are going to remove cow's milk from your child's diet it is important to provide an alternative such as soya milk as otherwise your child may lose weight. Don't remove all dairy products from your child's diet without trying to replace them with something else. You could give soya yogurt if your child cannot tolerate regular yogurt and choose a soya milk that is fortified with calcium.

Goat's and sheep's milk are not suitable for treating lactose intolerance as they contain lactose. If your child is still taking infant formula, it is possible to get lactose-free formulas which are very suitable for this purpose.

If your child's diarrhoea does not clear up when you remove lactose from the diet as above, consult your GP.

Be sure to re-introduce dairy products again after 4–6 weeks as otherwise your child may lose weight. If you do this and your child has diarrhoea again, you may need to ask your GP for further advice.

Constipation

Constipation is another common problem we see in children aged not only from 1–5 years but at any age from infancy to teens.

fluid intake for a child with constipation
Aim to give your child with constipation 6–8 cups of fluid a day including milk (1200 ml–1600 ml).

Constipation happens to almost everyone from time to time and is nothing to worry about. However, if it becomes ongoing or 'chronic', it can be very distressing for both the parents and the child.

For 90–95 per cent of children, the problem is 'functional' meaning it is not caused by a structural problem in the bowel or by any medical condition. It can be triggered by something as simple as having pain when passing a bowel motion. The child is then afraid to pass the next bowel motion, resulting in the stool becoming larger and even harder to pass. This can trigger off a chain of events that leads to chronic constipation.

Most children will grow out of constipation; however, it is important to seek medical advice if your child seems to be suffering from chronic constipation. Chronic constipation cannot be managed by diet alone. Your child may need to take medication for a while to help establish a normal pattern of going to the toilet again and to help them recognise when they need to go to the toilet.

Diet and constipation

The first thing to remember is that no one food or foods causes constipation, including milk or banana. However, certain foods certainly help treat or prevent constipation. Foods that help prevent constipation are those that contain fibre as it helps to make the stool bulkier allowing the gut to grab onto it and move it along better and more efficiently. Drinking adequate fluid is also very important in treating and preventing constipation.

Fluid Getting enough fluid in the diet helps to prevent stools from becoming dry and hard. If your child is suffering from constipation, the stools are probably already hard and drinking more fluid should help soften them.

The best type of fluid to give your child is water or milk. Soft drinks and juices may cause 'overflow diarrhoea'. Overflow diarrhoea is where your child is constipated but is having watery bowel motions that may stain underwear or bedclothes. What is happening is that a large stool is in the rectum but watery diarrhoea is building up behind it and leaking out. This can happen even if your child is not taking a lot of soft drinks or juices but it is still best to avoid them.

It is fine for your child to have one or two small cups of juice a day but do not allow any more juice than this. Aim to give about 600 ml (1 pint) of milk a day; the rest of the fluid intake should come from water.

Fibre is very important in both preventing and treating constipation. It works by trapping water in the stool to make it soften and by making the stool more bulky which helps it to move along the gut more efficiently. Fibre is also good for the overall health of the gut and may reduce the risk of colorectal cancer.

There are two types of fibre, soluble and insoluble. There is no need to be too concerned about the differences between the two but it is good to provide your child with a combination of the two.

While fibre is very good and should be a part of your child's diet, too much is not good for children as it may fill them up and stop them from eating other foods that provide important nutrients, for example calcium or iron. Too much fibre can also interfere with the absorption of other nutrients.

symptoms of chronic constipation
- Fewer than 3 bowel motions a week.
- Pain having a bowel motion.
- More than one episode of soiling a week.
- Large stools in the rectum that can be felt by the doctor when examining the abdomen.
- Behaviour that involves withholding stools.

two types of fibre
Soluble fibre is found in fruit, vegetables, oats, peas, beans and lentils.
Insoluble fibre is found in brown/whole meal bread, wholegrain cereals, pasta and crackers, brown rice and similar cereal-based foods.
A lot of fibre-containing foods contain both types of fibre.

How much fibre should I give my child?

There are no specific guidelines for children under 2 years of age. For children over 2 years, the American Health Foundation recommends 'age plus 5' g of fibre per day. In other words, a child aged 3 years should be having 3 + 5 = 8 g fibre per day.

compare the fibre content of some foods

	Food	Serving size	Fibre (g)
Breakfast cereals	Bran flakes	1 small bowl	4.0
	Weetabix	1 biscuit	2.5
	Rice krispies	1 small bowl	0.5
	Special K	1 small bowl	0.5
Breads	Wholemeal	1 large slice (38 g)	2.5
	Brown	1 large slice (35 g)	2.0
	White	1 large slice (30 g)	1.0
Fruit (fresh)	Apple	1 medium	1.5
	Banana	1 medium	1.0
	Grapes	1 small bunch	0.7
	Orange	1 medium	3.0
	Peach	1 medium	1.7
	Pear	1 medium	3.5
	Raspberries	7 medium	0.7
	Strawberries	7 medium	1.0
Fruit (dried)	Apricots	4 apricots	2.0
	Dates	2 dates	1.2
	Figs	1 fig	1.5
	Raisins	1 tablespoon	0.6
Vegetables	Broccoli, boiled	Small portion (60 g)	1.4
	Brussels sprouts, boiled	4 sprouts	1.0
	Cabbage	1 small portion (60 g)	1.0
	Cauliflower	6 florets (60 g)	1.0
	Carrot	1 medium (80 g)	2.0
	Cucumber	4 slices	0.1
	French beans	1 small potion (60g)	2.5
	Green pepper	2 rings	0.5
	Lettuce	4 leaves	0.5
	Potato, boiled	1 medium	0.7
	Potato, baked	1 small (including skin)	2.7
	Sweetcorn	1 tablespoon	0.5
	Tomato	1 small	1.0
Pulses	Baked beans	1 tablespoon	1.5
	Kidney beans	1 heaped tablespoon	2.3
	Peas	1 tablespoon	1.5
Pasta	White pasta	2 tablespoons	1.0
	Wholemeal pasta	2 tablespoons	2.0
Rice	Brown rice	2 tablespoons	1.0
	White rice	2 tablespoons	0.6
Cakes/scones	Fruit cake	1 slice	1.0
	Fruit scone	1 scone	1.0
	Wholemeal scone	1 scone	2.5
	Wholemeal cracker	2 crackers	0.8
	Digestive biscuit	1 biscuit	0.33

Aim to provide

- 2–5 portions of fruit and vegetables a day depending on age. Juice only counts as 1 portion no matter how many glasses are taken. It is always better to eat the whole fruit.
- A high-fibre cereal or porridge in the morning.
- 1 or 2 slices of whole meal bread throughout the day (1 for a younger toddler, 2 for an older toddler).

The following foods contain fibre and are good for your child if he or she is suffering from ongoing constipation.

Fibre-containing foods

- High fibre breakfast cereal. Look for one that has more than 6 g fibre per 100 g (this will be written on the nutritional label on the box).
- Whole meal bread.
- Whole meal crackers.
- Baked beans.
- Peas.
- Corn on the cob.
- Any type of vegetable, cooked or raw.
- Any type of fruit—raw or stewed. See page 125 for ideas on how to encourage your child to eat more fruit.)
- Raisins and other dried fruits.

What about fruit juice?

Fruit juice does not contain any fibre unless it has pulp. However, a fruit smoothie where the whole fruit has been blended contains fibre and can be a fun way to encourage your child to eat fruit.

Faltering growth

Growth in infancy is rapid—babies typically gain 6–7 kg (13–15½ lbs)during their first year. Thereafter this growth slows down and toddlers take on a leaner physique as they become more active. Children aged 1–5 years typically gain about 1–3 kg per year (2–6.5 lbs).

When a child is not gaining as much weight as expected doctors and health professionals may use the term 'faltering growth' to describe the condition. It can happen at any age from infancy to teens for various different reasons.

A toddler's growth may falter after an illness or illnesses or if the child is a fussy or restrictive eater. Growth faltering or poor weight gain can also be caused by an underlying illness or medical condition so it is very important to take your toddler to see your GP if you feel that weight gain is poor or the child has lost weight. Faltering growth can be serious if left untreated and can delay your child's development.

If your GP is happy, having seen your child, that there is no underlying condition causing the problem and your child just needs help with weight gain there are a number of approaches you can try. First, don't let your child go longer than 2–3 hours without eating. Toddlers are not able to eat a lot of food at one sitting so the best way to get more food into them over the day is to offer small amounts of food regularly. Offering 3 small meals and 3 snacks a day will help your child to eat more food overall. A glass of milk can be counted as part of a snack.

Good foods to help your child gain weight

- Full-fat milk, full fat yogurt and cheese
- Eggs (add a little butter and milk or cream to scrambled eggs or an omelette)
- Meat (can be fried in olive or vegetable oil for extra calories)
- Fish, especially oily fish such as salmon, trout and mackerel (again, fried)
- Avocados (one avocado contains almost 30 g fat)
- Pasta with creamy sauces such as spaghetti carbonara

Milk

Full-fat milk is a major source of calories, fat and protein for children and is particularly important if your child has poor weight gain. Aim to give your child 600 ml a day (3 glasses). Any more than this, however, may affect your child's appetite for solid food so it is probably better to stick to this amount. Milk can also be added to mashed potato, soup, cereal and anything else for extra calories (this does not need to be counted as part of the 600 ml a day). Older toddlers may take warm milk with some chocolate powder before bed.

'Addables' and 'spreadables'

If your child is not gaining weight it can be hard to simply give more food. You need to make sure that the small amounts of food that are eaten are high in calories. This is where 'addables' and 'spreadables' come in. These are high-calorie foods which can be added to or spread onto other foods to increase the calorie content of the meal or snack.

Spreadables	Addables
Butter	Cream
Margarine or spread (not low fat)	Oils such as olive oil or sunflower oil
Peanut butter (smooth)	Sour cream
Jam	Cheese
Honey	Crème fraîche
Mayonnaise	
Hummus	
Tahini	
Full-fat cream cheese	
Pesto	

This may strike you as not the healthiest list of foods in the world, with a few exceptions. However, if your child is failing to gain weight, you do not need to be concerned about the level of saturated fat in butter or cream. The only concern is that your child gains the necessary weight as that is the highest priority.

At the same time you should not give crisps, chips and chocolate all day long to get your child to gain weight. You are aiming to give the regular diet with extra sources of fat and calories added in to promote weight gain.

For example, 1 small bowl of tomato soup with 2 slices of unbuttered whole meal bread supply 315 calories but 1 small bowl of tomato soup with 2 tablespoons of cream added and 2 slices of generously buttered whole meal bread supply 500 calories.

How to incorporate 'addables' and 'spreadables' into your child's diet

- Add cream to cereal in the morning. If it is a cereal that is usually made up on water (e.g. porridge), make it up with milk instead and add cream.
- Spread butter and jam or honey on plain biscuits.
- Add cream to a tomato-based pasta sauce or a curry sauce.
- Add butter, milk and cream to mashed potatoes.
- Grate cheese onto pasta and potatoes.
- Offer mayonnaise as a dip with chips instead of ketchup or mix ketchup and mayonnaise together.
- Put peanut butter on toast or crackers.
- Drizzle melted butter or margarine on vegetables.
- Add a teaspoon of cream into a yogurt.
- Grate cheese into mashed dinners.
- Use mayonnaise/grated cheese/salad cream/hummus in sandwiches.
- Try two fillings, such as ham and cheese, in sandwiches.

If your child does not gain enough weight seek advice from a qualified dietitian. See www.indi.ie for a list of qualified dietitians working in your area or ask your GP or local health centre if there is a dietitian you can see.

12 Dealing with food refusal

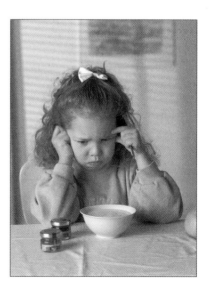

Many parents and carers report that one of the hardest and most frustrating aspects of child rearing is 'feeding the kids'. Young children are developing their own personalities and temperaments and in some cases food refusal is their way of exerting their independence or commanding attention.

Most of the problems associated with children refusing food develop because parents worry and give the child too much attention for *not* eating. So try not to be concerned if your child is refusing food. It is probably just a temporary thing and most children go through a phase of not eating.

However, the nutritional requirements of a child are very high relative to size and making sure a child obtains enough nutrition can be very difficult if he or she seems to be refusing all the wholesome meals and snacks being offered.

Distractions at meal times, poor routine, excessive intake of drinks, limited variety of food, inappropriate weaning, not to mention manipulative behaviour or parental anxiety, all contribute to food refusal or 'fussy eating'.

In this chapter we focus on child-centred strategies that will direct rather than control your child. However, you will need to be consistent in your approach. By applying the following recommendations you will be doing all you can to ensure your child learns to enjoy and eat the wholesome diet you provide.

How to identify if your child is eating poorly

First of all, ask yourself if this is just one of those days where your child is not eating well but you know he or she will eat better tomorrow. If this is the case then there is nothing to worry about. It is normal for toddlers to eat very little one day and lots the next day.

However, if you feel that your child has been eating poorly for a number of days or weeks but does not seem unwell in any way and has plenty of energy, try writing down everything your child eats and drinks for a number of days. It could be that the child is in fact eating quite a lot of small things over the course of the day and that this adds up to more than you thought.

If you write down everything that your child is eating and it still seems like very little check if he or she is drinking a lot of juice, cordial or soft drink, even milk, over the day that may be taking away the appetite.

Drinks

A child's stomach capacity is much smaller than an adult's. If a child drinks excessively before meals, or randomly throughout the day, appetite will be significantly reduced. Children sometimes choose to fill up on drinks instead of eating their meals. In our experience this is the most common cause of poor appetite in children. We often see children who have been drinking up to 2 litres of juice per day (10 glasses) and don't have enough space left in their stomach for food! Therefore we strongly urge parents to take control of the type, amount and timing of drinks.

case study: Emily, aged 18 months

Emily attended our clinic because her parents were worried that she wasn't eating enough. Meal times were a battle as Emily didn't seem hungry for food and it was a struggle to get her to eat even a tiny portion of a meal. She liked milk and was drinking nearly 2 litres of growing-up milk a day. She was growing normally and wasn't underweight but was quite constipated. Emily was basically filling up on milk which left no room in her diet for other foods. The growing-up milk was providing Emily with all the calories, protein and iron that she needed to grow properly. However, the lack of solid foods in her diet meant that Emily wasn't developing her feeding skills and wasn't eating enough fibre. Her parents were advised to limit her milk intake to 600 mls a day and after just a couple of weeks Emily was eating much better and learning new feeding skills.

case study: Conor, aged 2 years

Conor attended our clinic because he was a little bit underweight for his height. He was a picky eater and although he was 2 years old he was still drinking from a baby bottle. He was a busy, active child, always on the go. He loved drinking squash and diluted juice from his bottle and his parents had to fill the bottle several times a day. Although the squash and diluted juice were low in calories, they were filling up his small tummy and taking the edge off his appetite for food. Small children find drinking from a baby bottle much easier than an open cup. A bottle is also easy for them to carry around and allows them to take frequent drinks while playing. Conor's parents were advised to throw away his bottle and to offer all drinks from an open cup. They were also advised to offer water instead of juice and not to give any drinks before meals. Conor was very upset initially but within a few weeks he had forgotten his bottle, was drinking a lot less squash and diluted juice and was eating much better.

When your baby is 6 months old you should introduce a cup or beaker for drinks. Discourage feeding from a bottle after the age of 1 year.

If your child is drinking juice, limit it to 1 or 2 small glasses a day and don't allow any drinks for up to half an hour before meals. You should not need to restrict your child's intake of water unless he or she is drinking a lot right before meals. Try to avoid giving your toddler soft drinks completely except on special occasions.

Children over 1 year old should drink no more than 600 mls (1 pint) of fresh milk daily. If you are concerned that your child is drinking too much milk measure out a pint of milk, leave it in the fridge and use only this amount of milk each day. Many parents are reluctant to reduce their child's milk intake, naturally feeling that the only nourishment their child is getting is from milk. However, it is a necessary first step. Milk is a poor source of iron and drinking too much will reduce the amount of food eaten which often leads to constipation as well as iron-deficiency anaemia.

Drinking too much liquid can lessen your child's appetite; so you should limit liquid consumption to 3–4 cups daily plus the 600 mls of milk, maximum 1200–1500 mls per day. This will ensure your child is hungry enough to eat solid foods. Bear in mind that if your child has a good intake of other dairy foods, such as cheese and yogurt, over the day there will be no need to take 600 mls every day to meet calcium needs.

Try to avoid giving fizzy drinks because they are very filling. It is best to avoid buying them altogether. Make a house rule of no drinks for 30 minutes before meals. Limit drinks at mealtimes to half a cup of water (120 mls) and ensure that at least half the meal is eaten before allowing the drink.

dos and don'ts when giving drinks to children over 1 year old

- Don't give fizzy drinks.
- Do give 600 mls (1 pint) of milk plus 3–4 cups of other liquid a day.
- Don't give drinks for 30 minutes before a meal.
- Don't give more than half a cup of water during a meal, and don't give it until half the meal is eaten.

Have regular mealtimes

Keep mealtimes regular and familiar. Children thrive on routine; it gets them into a rhythm of eating which revolves around set mealtimes during the day.

Offer 3 main meals at around the same time every day with 2–3 snacks spaced in between, depending on age. This makes meals significant events and helps children to learn that a main meal is not just another snack or sideshow that can easily be taken or left. Meals are occasions to be enjoyed while socialising with the family, household members or friends. Established mealtimes may actually make it easier for the family (adults and children) to eat together more often.

A good meal routine programmes hunger or appetite. If your child eats meals at the same times every day his or her appetite will adapt and be trained to feel hungry at mealtimes.

Snacks

Toddlers and young children need to eat more often than an older child. Small scheduled snacks, spaced between meals are usually necessary 2–3 times a day. For most, peak snack time is mid afternoon. However, a string of snacks, nibbles or drinks randomly throughout the day leaves children never fully satisfied or hungry. If children are allowed to snack all day long on sweet or salty snack foods, for example biscuits or crisps, they will happily comply and refuse their main meals.

Tips for happy eating

- Have meals at the same time every day.
- Eat together as a family as much as possible.
- Place your child at the table in a suitable seat.
- Finish your own meal before helping your child.
- Don't let your child drink more than 600 mls of milk and 3–4 cups of other fluid a day—on average 1200–1400 mls in total per day.
- Try not to react if your child refuses to eat his or her meal.
- Minimise distractions such as television, open doors etc., during meals.
- Let your child play with food, and encourage self-feeding.
- Don't allow unlimited snacking throughout the day.
- Vary the food you serve to older children — they get bored with the same food all the time.

Eating together

Make the meal table a relaxed and positive environment, free of family conflict, tensions and distractions (such as television). Whenever possible allow your child to eat with the rest of the family. Children watch how adults eat and we can expect that they too in time will do the same. Family mealtimes offer a terrific opportunity to teach children good eating patterns.

Serve both adults and children at the same time. Children learn through observation and their natural desire to copy. You should finish your own meal before helping or prompting your child with his or her meal. Adults must remain the focus of attention during the meal. This will make the child more curious about what's on his or her own plate.

Avoid letting your child eat off your or another adult's plate, especially when adults and children have similar food on their plates. Minimise distraction during meals by switching off the television, closing doors and removing toys. Provide suitable seating at an appropriate height for the table. Discourage your child from eating while walking or standing.

Eat something yourself with your child—even just a small amount is worthwhile, if you are planning to eat your meal later. Meals are better fun if there is someone to share with.

The menu

Food preferences are all about familiarity of taste and experiences. Babies are born with a natural preference for sweet-tasting foods and have to learn to like other flavours. Children learn to like the food they are regularly exposed to. There is evidence that exposure to tastes increases food acceptance.

Except for the early stages of weaning, it is vital to prepare the same menu for both adults and children. The child will feel enticed to try what everyone else is eating and this will help to introduce variety into his or her diet.

Offer one new food at a time, as a small portion (initially this can be as small as a teaspoon). Serve the unfamiliar food with familiar ones.

Don't be put off by food rejection. You may need to offer an individual food repeatedly (this could be up to 14 times—don't expect acceptance for the first 10 times in many cases) before the food looks familiar or the taste is acquired and your child chooses to eat it. Unfortunately, a lot of parents persist only two or three times before giving up on a particular food altogether, or presume that if something is refused today it will be refused for life.

Abandon presentation gimmicks such as potato waffles or chicken nuggets in animal shapes or the equivalent. Children may like the idea of them but not actually eat more and you may find yourself on a permanent quest for new and novel ways of presenting their food.

Offer easy-to-eat foods by cutting up large items that can be eaten with fingers. Children eat better if they are allowed to feed themselves, and are not spoon fed. This will mean your babies and toddlers are covered in food after every meal, and you won't be able to hurry through mealtimes, but it will be worth it. There is a strong link between allowing your child to have fun with food and willingness to try new tastes and textures.

Introduce texture gradually from 6 months of age. It is important to progress from purées to minced or mashed dinners with soft lumps and to offer your child soft finger foods by roughly 9 months of age.

Delaying your baby's exposure to lumpier foods may contribute to fussy eating and food refusal. 'Lumpy foods' are semi-solids such as bits of cooked soft vegetables or food that is semi-puréed. It does not mean hard foods that could be a choking hazard.

Once teeth develop children tend to appreciate foods that have some bite before disintegrating in the mouth. Try serving pasta shapes, boiled egg, pieces of meat, baked beans, for example.

Don't pile food on the plate. Serve individual foods as small portions that are separated, not touching each other on their plate. This enables your child to identify the food and its flavour and texture. Children usually eat better when the portions are small.

When choosing food for meal times remember younger children may never tire of the few foods they especially like while older children get progressively bored with eating the same foods.

Children do not automatically have the sophisticated taste of adults; so some reasonable compromise needs to be made when sharing the same menu.

Remember to keep it simple. Once children are happily taking a variety of foods you can introduce dishes such as quiche and richer foods, as you wish.

Fussy eating

Food refusal is a huge phenomenon. All children refuse to eat their meals at times and some children regularly refuse to eat. However, most adults overestimate and generalise children's food dislikes, almost accepting fussiness as normal or expected.

when do I need to worry about my child not eating or drinking?

If fluids (drinks) are being refused then you should consult your GP as it is possible your child is unwell. Children are quite susceptible to dehydration so if they are not drinking, seek medical advice. Similarly if your child is not eating and seems unwell or 'out of sorts', it is important that you bring him or her to your GP or local A & E.

multivitamin and mineral supplements

If your child's diet is very limited or the fussy eating continues, it is no harm to give him or her a multivitamin and mineral supplement, for example, Vivioptal Junior (liquid), Forceval Junior (capsule) or Centrum Junior (tablet). Check individual dosage for age as recommended by the manufacturer.

Always consult your pharmacist before you buy a supplement, as not all supplements are suitable for children.

Never let your child hear you talking about how fussy he or she is as there is no doubt that a child can choose to be fussy as a form of attention seeking. Don't allow your frustration to become obvious either. Stay calm (in front of the child at least) and positive.

When dealing with children who say 'no', don't resort to force-feeding or bribery. Force-feeding pays no dividends. Instead it creates a strong negative association with food that the child will remember. Bribery teaches children that eating is a chore they have to face in order to have something more pleasant. Despite being very tempting, resist this in all circumstances. Adopting bribery as a tactic to persuade children to eat hands them ammunition to use against their parents and once they realise it works they won't hesitate to use it.

Remember not to underestimate your child's IQ or perception. Most children work out that if they refuse to eat their meal, adults will eventually give in. This will set a precedent that adults do not really mean what they say. Therefore if your child refuses to eat a meal do not offer an alternative meal or snack.

Toddlers especially can be exceptionally stubborn when refusing food and will not give in, even resorting to such melodramatic acts as falling off the chair or vomiting to avoid eating their food. At this stage it would be understandable if you lost your cool only to regret it later. Avoid making mealtimes a battle of wills. Keep calm. Simply remove uneaten food without comment at the end of the meal; do not insist on a clean plate. Set a time limit for mealtime, such as 30 minutes.

Providing growth is satisfactory and there is no physiological cause for loss of appetite, children are unlikely to come to any harm with a few missed meals. If your child doesn't eat much at one meal, he or she will probably eat more at the next.

Children will not allow themselves to go hungry and by refraining from offering a substitute or a snack they will learn it's best to eat their dinner. This will not happen after one episode. Persistence is required.

Undoubtedly tantrums will occur, but they will be short lived if you stay consistent in your approach.

It is important to assess your own response to your child's refusal of food. Children crave attention and often don't mind what type they get. Therefore the less attention given to a negative situation the better. By contrast, load on the attention to a positive situation. Give lots of praise, hugs, and kisses (not rewards) even if a small quantity of food is eaten.

Just like adults, children should be allowed to have certain food dislikes. Decide together what can be left out for the time being. Let your child choose three or four specific foods that can be left out of meals, but not whole food groups. For example, it's all right to dislike broccoli but it's not acceptable to dislike all vegetables. If you follow this approach your child will feel listened to and be more open to trying new foods.

Avoid placing food into categories of 'good' and 'bad' and discussing food dislikes in front of children.

Don't ignore problems that interfere with eating such as teething, sore throat, blocked nose or an upset tummy.

Children tend to eat up if they are allowed to serve themselves and help in the meal preparation process. Little ones can set the table, call everyone to the table or time the cooking with an egg timer.

Peer modelling is very helpful. Children enjoy eating with other children and you can encourage this, especially if the others eat a varied diet. Occasionally change the venue, for example, to a picnic.

Remember to be a good role model. Eat a wide variety of foods yourself.

do
- Encourage and praise your child when he or she eats well.
- Allow your child to have dislikes and likes.
- Pay attention to problems that interfere with eating — colds, etc.
- Stay calm — in face of all provocation!

don't
- Make mealtimes a battle of wills.
- Bribe your child to eat.
- Force-feed your child.
- Offer alternatives if your child refuses to eat a meal.
- Discuss food issues in front of your child.

Food and growth

Children's appetite usually adjusts itself to the amount and type of food that provides the energy that they need to live and grow. What's most important to the child's health and growth is not the quantity, but the quality of the food eaten.

One of the most important indicators of whether there is a serious feeding problem is your child's overall growth pattern. If your child, like other healthy children, is growing and gaining weight normally he or she is most likely to be in good health and does not have a serious feeding problem. The public health nurse, practice nurse or GP will be able to check weight and growth rate and confirm that it fits the normal pattern.

It is worth visiting your GP if the dietary intake is consistently poor or weight loss is noticed and growth is static. Your GP will review overall weight gain and growth progress, take a history of bowel movements and general well being, and may take a blood test to rule out iron-deficiency anaemia.

If you are concerned about anything you should seek the advice of a paediatric dietitian who will carry out a detailed dietary assessment and make a comparison with the nutritional targets for the relevant age and circumstance. Dietary intervention and advice will be tailored to your child's specific requirements and food preferences. The GP will refer your child to the community dietitian if there is one practising in the area. Unfortunately, at present there are not many community dietitians employed to provide a paediatric service and not all hospital paediatric dietitians can accept referrals from GPs.

seeing a dietitian privately

If you would like to see a dietitian privately the best way to find one with paediatric experience is to visit the website of the Irish Nutrition and Dietetic Institute (INDI) at www.indi.ie or telephone (01) 280 4839 (9.30 a.m. to 12.30 p.m.). The INDI is the professional body for dietitians in Ireland.

Using the combination of practical measures and behavioural techniques discussed in this chapter should result in the majority of fussy eaters growing normally and without nutritional deficiencies.

Fussy eating is not uncommon; many children are difficult to feed especially during their early years. If, despite your best efforts, your child is still very fussy about food intake, concentrate in particular on sharing the same menu for the whole family and eating together as much as possible. Be prepared to give plenty of gentle encouragement. Finally, and most importantly, do not doubt your ability as a good parent.

Food allergy

13

Nearly 4.5% or 1 in 22 five-year-olds in Ireland have a food allergy to egg, peanut, other nut or milk (Cork Baseline Study 2016). Food allergy is a sometimes dangerous form of unpleasant reaction to food. While food allergy can develop at any age, it is most commonly diagnosed before the age of 3 years. Fortunately, up to 90 per cent of children grow out of their food allergy by the time they are 6 years old.

If you suspect that your child may have a food allergy, a correct diagnosis is essential and expert medical advice should be sought. Paediatric allergy services aim to improve the quality of life for children with food allergy, allowing children to live, play and be educated without restrictions and stigmatisation. The website www.ifan.ie provides excellent information on diagnosing and managing food allergy. A new section on the website specifically for parents is currently under development and should become available in the near future. Hopefully, in time, through the lobbying action of such groups as the Irish Food Allergy Network (IFAN) and individual parents, all children with food allergies throughout Ireland will have access to expert medical care when and where they need it most.

While living with a severe food allergy can be a constant source of worry, it is important for both children and families to participate in normal social activities as much as possible.

In this chapter we advise on how best to cope with your child's food allergy. If your baby is at high risk of developing a food allergy we advise what steps to take to try to prevent this occurring.

top 6 foods causing allergic reactions in children in Ireland and the UK

- Hen's egg
- Tree nuts
- Fish
- Peanut
- Cow's milk
- Shellfish

Note Fish or shellfish allergy is rare in younger children; most cases are diagnosed in late teens and early 20s.

Food aversion, intolerance & allergy

It is important to distinguish between food aversion, food intolerance and food allergy—all are unpleasant reactions to food but they have different causes and consequences.

Food aversion

With food aversion the type of unpleasant reaction to a food is psychological e.g. if a child has a tummy bug and the last food he or she ate before the vomiting started was cheese, the child may now associate cheese with vomiting. Cheese will be avoided, at least for a while, as the thought of eating it makes the child feel sick. However, if the cheese is hidden and the child is not aware of having eaten it, an unpleasant reaction does not occur!

Food intolerance

Food intolerance is a type of food hypersensitivity which provokes an unpleasant reaction. It may be caused by an enzyme deficiency or disorder of protein metabolism or a reaction to a chemical present in a food. Food intolerance may last a few weeks or it may last a lifetime.

An example of food intolerance is intolerance to lactose, the naturally occurring sugar in milk. Lactase, an important digestive enzyme in the gut, is needed to digest lactose but sometimes levels are reduced, for example after severe gastroenteritis. As a consequence the baby or young child is unable to digest lactose and has diarrhoea. The lactase levels will return to normal after 6 to 8 weeks. For more information on lactose intolerance see pages 110–111 and 155–6.

Food allergy

Food allergy is another type of food sensitivity causing an unpleasant reaction to food. The crucial difference between food allergy and food intolerance is that in allergy the unpleasant reaction is caused by the body's immune system. Food allergy occurs when the body's immune system reacts to a food as if it isn't safe. In the same way that the immune system fights off bacteria and viruses, the immune systems reacts against a food. It is the protein component of a food that triggers the reaction. Put simply, food allergy is a failure to tolerate certain key food proteins.

If someone has a severe food allergy the reaction can be life threatening. This very severe form of reaction associated with food allergy is called anaphylaxis (pronounced anna-fill-axis).

food aversion, intolerance and allergy

Food aversion
- Causes an unpleasant reaction to a food.
- Has a psychological component.
- Makes the child feel ill (only if aware the food has been eaten).

Food intolerance
- Causes an unpleasant reaction to a food.
- Is a type of food sensitivity.
- Makes the child feel ill.

Food allergy
- Causes an unpleasant reaction to a food.
- Is a type of food sensitivity.
- Makes the child feel ill.
- Involves the immune system.

Common food allergens

All over the world a limited number of foods are responsible for the majority of food-induced allergic reactions. However, it is possible for any food that contains protein to trigger an allergic reaction. Even foods with tiny amounts of protein such as kiwi fruit, mango, rice and potato have been known to cause allergic reactions. In the UK allergy to kiwi fruit is becoming more common. In France common food allergens include snail, mustard seed and lentils and in Spain allergy to peach is common.

There is a high recovery rate for most food allergies except peanuts, tree nuts, fish and shellfish. While there is a much poorer recovery rate for peanuts, it is estimated that up to 20 per cent of children with peanut allergy may outgrow it.

Symptoms of food allergy

Food allergy symptoms are usually caused by eating the food. In milder cases it may be possible to eat a small amount of the food without having a reaction. This is known as having a 'threshold' or 'dose response' to a food, where it takes a certain amount of the food to trigger the allergic reaction. However, in severe cases of food allergy symptoms are caused by eating the tiniest amounts of the food.

None or only very mild symptoms will be caused by touching or smelling the food, for example, skin contact by kissing somebody who has just eaten the food or inhalation of cooking fumes or tiny particles of food in the air.

Food allergic reactions can affect the skin, gut, lungs or heart/blood pressure. Children can be affected differently. Different children who are allergic to the same food may not experience the same reaction to that food. Reactions can vary from mild to a life-threatening medical emergency (anaphylaxis). For example, where two children have a milk allergy, one child may suffer from hives following accidental milk ingestion whereas the other child may have an anaphylactic reaction.

In addition, the child's reaction to the food may not always be the same. This is a very important point to remember, particularly if an allergy to nuts or seeds is suspected. It is impossible to predict the future course of reactions based on previous reactions. Always seek medical advice as soon as possible following a first reaction to nuts or seeds.

On the other hand, while a child usually begins to have symptoms after the first exposure to a food, this is not always the case. Sometimes food allergic reaction develops over time.

Allergic reactions that affect the skin only are classed as mild. The most severe form of allergic reaction, anaphylaxis, can affect the body's airways, blood circulation and heart.

Diagnosing food allergy

If you suspect that your child has a food allergy it is best to consult your GP or health professional. If he or she is not experienced in dealing with food allergy your child may be referred to a paediatrician or allergy specialist. The diagnosis should be made as early as possible. (See page 194–5 for names and addresses of doctors who specialise in the treatment of allergy.)

An allergy focused clinical history and food challenges are two important components of making an accurate diagnosis. No single laboratory test can diagnose food allergy. Some forms of allergy can be tested for but the results of the test do not by themselves confirm or exclude allergy.

Swift or delayed allergic reaction to a food

The symptoms experienced during an allergic reaction may occur within 2 hours of eating the food or may be delayed for 24 hours or longer. The longer the length of time between eating a food and developing symptoms means it's hard to see the connection between the two.

Where the reaction is fairly immediate diagnosis is somewhat easier than in cases where the reaction is delayed. This is because the allergic reactions happen in one of two ways.

Allergic reactions are either:

- *IgE (Immunoglobulin E)-mediated:* symptoms appear usually within 2 hours (and often within minutes) of eating a small amount of the food, or
- *Non-IgE-mediated:* symptoms may not occur for up to 24 hours or longer (in some cases up to 3 days) after eating the food.

The distinction between the two ways of experiencing food allergy is important because there are tests available to guide diagnosis and management of swift (IgE-mediated allergic) reactions but there is none for delayed (non IgE-mediated allergic) reactions. To guide the diagnosis and management of non IgE-mediated allergic reactions an elimination diet followed by the reintroduction of excluded foods will be necessary. Elimination diets should only be undertaken under the supervision of a registered dietitian, should exclude no more than four foods and should last no longer than 4–6 weeks.

IgE (Immunoglobulin) is an antibody. Antibodies are immune cells that circulate in the bloodstream ready to destroy any harmful substance (bacteria, viruses) that may enter the body. IgE is a specific antibody associated with food allergies. In an IgE-mediated allergic reaction the body inappropriately produces lots of IgE antibodies against the food protein.

Tests for food allergic reactions

There are two methods for checking for IgE antibodies—the skin prick test (SPT) and the Specific IgE test.

Both IgE and non-IgE-mediated food allergy should be properly treated and investigated by a multidisciplinary health care team including paediatrician/allergy specialist, dietitian and nurse.

symptoms of food allergy

Skin Itchy skin; rash, hives; swelling of the lips and tongue.

Gut Nausea and feeling bloated; diarrhoea and/or vomiting; reflux.

Lung/chest Itchy, runny or blocked nose; coughing; hoarseness; wheezing; shortness of breath.

Heart/blood pressure Faintness and collapse.

Other Sore, red and itchy eyes; dry, itchy throat.

warning

There is neither a rational scientific basis nor proven role for hair analysis, isolated IgG testing, Kinesiology, Vega testing or Enzyme Potentiated Desensitization for diagnosing or managing food allergy. These tests are simply a waste of time, not to mention money.

allergic symptoms associated with asthma

■ **Food-induced wheezing** Approximately 6 per cent of children with asthma have food-induced wheezing. If you suspect that your child's asthma is affected by certain foods you should ask your doctor to refer you to an allergy specialist.

■ **Allergic rhinitis** is an allergic response to either wind-borne pollens or grasses, trees and weeds or house dust mite allergens, pet dander and mould spores. It affects up to 80 per cent of asthmatic children. Symptoms include chronic recurrent sneezing, nasal congestion, clear runny nasal secretions and itchy nose, eyes, soft palate and ears. Proper treatment of rhinitis in children who have asthma improves their asthma. To receive proper treatment for rhinitis it may be necessary for your child to attend an allergy specialist.

■ **Egg allergy and the chances of developing asthma** A child with egg allergy, especially if it is diagnosed before 1 year of age, has a much higher risk of developing asthma when he or she is older than a child without egg allergy.

■ **Eczema and food allergy** Children under 1 year of age who have both eczema and a food allergy, have a high risk of developing asthma by 5 years of age.

Skin prick test (SPT)

With this test, different types of food extract are put on tiny areas of scratched skin. A drop of food extract is put on the skin and then the skin is pricked with a small needle through the drop. The test can also be done with a pricking device that has been presoaked in food extract. Only the top layer of the skin is pricked and the test does not draw any blood. The test is usually done on the back or arm. The skin test is ready to check in about 15 minutes.

A red bump or weal that looks like a mosquito bite will appear at the spot where the food extract was placed. Your doctor or health professional will measure the size of the weal. The size indicates whether the test result is positive or not. The weal will disappear within an hour.

A skin prick test can be carried out on babies of any age.

If your child has been taking anti-histamines the skin prick will have to be delayed. The type of anti-histamine dictates the length of time that needs to elapse between stopping taking it and a skin prick test. For children liquid anti-histamines are recommended as the syrups are absorbed more quickly than tablets.

IgE-mediated symptoms

Rash/hives; swelling of lips and tongue; nausea; abdominal pain; vomiting; diarrhoea; itchy/runny nose; itchy, red eyes; breathing difficulties.

non-IgE-mediated symptoms

Diarrhoea; reflux; constipation.

Name of anti-histamine	Time lapse needed between stopping anti-histamine and SPT
Piriton	48 hours
Zirteck	1 week
Clarity	1 week
Hismanal	1 month

Note It is very important if your child has an allergic reaction prior to their appointment for skin prick testing to give them their prescribed anti-histamine. The appointment for the skin prick testing can be rescheduled.

Specific IgE test (SpIgE)

SpIgE has replaced an older type of test called RAST. It is a blood test measuring the amount of IgE antibody in the blood. It is not necessary for the child to stop taking anti-histamines before the test. The results show whether a child is making antibody to the foods tested for and thus is sensitised to these foods. It usually takes a couple of weeks for the test results to come back.

Assessing the results of SPT and SpIgE tests

These tests do not give a definite answer about the presence of an allergy. The results are more like betting odds, indicating the likelihood of having an allergic reaction to a particular food. A diagnosis of food allergy cannot be made on the basis of the SPT or SpIgE test results alone.

If your child has a positive test result to egg, and also has a positive medical history, e.g. every time he or she eats egg a rash and facial swelling develop, then this is usually sufficient to confirm a diagnosis of egg allergy.

If your child has a positive test result to peanut but has no medical history of reacting to peanut, then further tests such as a food challenge are needed. The SPT and SpIgE are not 100 per cent reliable and sometimes results can be falsely positive or falsely negative.

If your child has a positive medical history, e.g. eczema always worsens after eating yogurts or other dairy foods, but the SPT or SpIgE test for milk is negative, he or she may have a non IgE-mediated food allergy. As mentioned earlier the SPT and SpIgE can only detect IgE-mediated food allergy. They are of no use when it comes to checking for non-IgE-mediated food allergy.

allergy tests

An allergy focused clinical history is an important part of diagnosing food allergy. Two key questions your doctor or health professional will ask concern the length of time that passes between your child eating a food and developing a reaction and the symptoms involved. If the suspected food contains more than one ingredient you will need to provide a list of all the ingredients in the food.

Following the medical history, your doctor or health professional will decide which tests, if any, might be indicated and which foods need to be tested.

Test results do not predict the severity of allergic reactions. It is simply not possible to know how allergic a child is to a food. Allergic reactions are unpredictable and may vary in severity from one occasion to the next.

Note Expert medical opinion is crucial in obtaining an accurate diagnosis and the safest treatment possible for your child.

Food challenge

Following SPT and SpIgE tests a food challenge may be undertaken, depending on your child's medical history. For example, your doctor or healthcare professional would never ask a child who had a positive SpIgE result to peanut and has a history of a severe allergic reaction to peanut to undertake a food challenge as part of the diagnosis. However children are sometimes offered food challenges to give them the opportunity to experience a reaction and know what it feels like.

During a food challenge, gradually increasing amounts of a food are given to the child, while the doctor or health care professional watches for symptoms. Usually every 15–30 minutes the child is given an increasing dose of the suspected food allergen, and is then closely observed for any signs of a reaction. This test should only be done by a trained professional who is ready to treat your child in the event of a serious reaction to the food.

As mentioned earlier, up to 90 per cent of children grow out of their food allergy by 6 years of age. The prognosis of childhood food allergy is good, with the exception of peanuts, tree nuts, fish and sea food.

As part of your child's ongoing treatment for food allergy, food challenges may be repeated over time to avoid unnecessarily prolonged avoidance diets.

Any food challenges should always be discussed with your doctor or healthcare professional first as the child's clinical history and test results will need to be taken into consideration. Depending on the severity of the food allergy, food challenges may need to be done in hospital. In milder cases it may be possible to do the challenge at home, provided your doctor or healthcare professional has advised that it is safe to do so.

Up to 20 per cent of children with peanut allergy may actually outgrow their allergy so food challenges should also be considered for this group of children.

Children who are losing their allergies (developing tolerance) or are outgrowing them, may continue to have positive SPT and SpIgE results for a number of years after their symptoms have disappeared.

Elimination diets

In cases of delayed allergic reactions (non-IgE-mediated symptoms), it can be very difficult to make a diagnosis of food allergy. Sometimes the only option may be to remove the suspected food or foods from the child's diet for a period of up to 4 to 6 weeks and monitor symptoms for any signs of improvement.

Elimination diets should only be undertaken under the supervision of a registered dietitian, should exclude no more than four foods and should last no longer than 4–6 weeks. Children on restricted diets are very vulnerable to developing nutritional deficiencies and it is important that any child on such a diet receives a detailed dietary assessment and is monitored regularly to ensure the diet is nutritionally adequate.

It is also crucial that if a food is being removed from the diet, all sources of the food, including hidden sources, are removed. For example, what do some flavoured crisps, muesli and chocolate have in common? The answer is they all contain cow's milk protein! Without removing all sources of a food from the diet, it is impossible to tell whether or not a child has an allergy to that food.

Your GP or doctor can refer you to a dietitian. If it is not possible for you to see a hospital or community dietitian see page 195 for how to find a registered dietitian working in private practice in your area.

Eczema and food allergy

Eczema is a major disease in children, usually developing before two years of age, and it can be a very debilitating illness. The cause of eczema is complex and not fully understood. Foods are not the single cause or cure of eczema. Defects in skin barrier function have a major role to play. There is no cure—the aim of treatment is the control of symptoms.

As a parent it is easy to look to diet as a potential treatment for your child's eczema. Diet can seem an easy thing to change and it allows you to feel that you are able to do something to help your child. However, food allergy as a cause of eczema is very unusual. Skin care should always be fully optimised before removing foods from your child's diet. While food allergy is a very uncommon cause of eczema, children with moderate to severe eczema are at higher risk of developing food allergy. Up to 84% of babies who develop moderate to severe eczema before three months of age will have food allergies. In these high risk infants it is advisable to test for egg and nut allergy before starting solids. Foods can exacerbate eczema but when these children stop eating the foods they are allergic to, most of them still have some eczema and will need to continue their skin care routine.

It is not easy to diagnose suspected food allergy in eczema. Most children with allergies to food may develop worse eczema and a hive-like reaction immediately or within two hours after eating a food and become very itchy. The most commonly offending foods are eggs, dairy, nuts and wheat. If you suspect your child may have a food allergy, it can help to keep a food and symptoms diary and show this to your doctor. Never remove any foods from your child's diet without consulting your doctor first. Your doctor will be able to refer you to an allergy specialist if necessary.

Children excluding staple foods from their diets such as dairy and wheat can quickly develop nutritional deficiencies leading to malnutrition, and this type of diet should only be undertaken if your doctor is in agreement and an experienced paediatric dietitian is available to supervise and manage the diet.

Dietary treatment will not cure a child's eczema but it may improve the symptoms.

A good skin care routine will remain a vital part of care. The Royal Children's Hospital in Melbourne has produced an excellent booklet for parents called 'Knowing Your Child's Eczema'. To download a free copy of the booklet visit the ifan.ie website and click on the link 'knowing your child's eczema'. The National Eczema Society in the UK is also a very good source of information. Comprehensive downloads on emollients and steroids are available from the Society's website, eczema.org.

If your child has significant eczema which is not responding well to treatment and especially if he or she is under 2 years old, you should speak to your GP regarding a referral to a paediatrican/dermatologist for expert assessment.

living with a food allergy can be very difficult for families. Depending on the severity of the allergic reaction, constant vigilance may be required to ensure the child does not accidentally eat a food to which he or she is allergic. This can cause tremendous stress and strain to the whole family. The dietitian's main role is to help families adapt their food and eating so they can live as normal a life as possible. It is important that children with food allergies are not socially excluded from parties and sleepovers.

Referral to a dietitian following diagnosis of a food allergy

All children with a food allergy should be seen by an experienced paediatric dietitian. The dietitian will be able to provide you with the most up to date information available and offer education and support as necessary, while at the same time ensuring your child continues to receive an adequate dietary intake of all nutrients in a safe way. He or she will provide practical advice on shopping, cooking, recipes, cost issues, prescription items, product information and nutritional supplements. A general discussion around menu planning is helpful!

Ideally a child with a severe or potentially severe food allergy should be seen by a dietitian within 2 weeks of diagnosis. The initial appointment should be followed by a review appointment approximately 6 weeks later. Children should be seen by their dietitian a minimum of once a year and more frequently if needed. Children's nutritional needs change with time and it is essential that their growth and nutrient intake is monitored at least once a year especially if staple foods such as milk and wheat have to be excluded from the diet.

Anaphylaxis

Anaphylaxis is the medical term for a severe allergic reaction that affects the whole body. In its most extreme form, the reaction can result in the person going into 'anaphylactic shock' which can be fatal.

Anaphylaxis to food is not uncommon. However fatal food induced anaphylaxis is extremely rare. In the UK, between 2000 and 2006, 11 children died due to food allergic reactions. Almost all the children had a previous history of food allergy. As mentioned earlier it is impossible to predict how allergic a child is going to be to a food and in the case of allergy to nuts and seeds medical advice should be sought as soon as possible following the first reaction.

The following foods are the most common cause of anaphylaxis: peanuts, tree nuts, fish (especially shellfish) and sesame seeds. Wasp or bee stings, natural latex (rubber), penicillin and other drugs can also cause anaphylaxis. It is estimated that peanut allergy may affect as many as 16,000 children in Ireland.

Poorly controlled asthma is another significant risk factor for the development of food anaphylaxis. Severe wheeze is a prominent feature of severe allergic reactions and therefore needs the very best medical management. All children with both asthma and a food allergy should attend an allergy specialist for assessment and advice. About 6 per cent of children with asthma have food-induced wheezing.

Symptoms of anaphylaxis

Symptoms of anaphylaxis include tingling sensation of the lips, tongue and throat, pallor, swelling of the lips, mouth or tongue, dry 'staccato' or barking cough—young children may just scratch at the tongue, roof of the mouth or throat—swelling of the throat, wheezing, difficulty breathing, drop in blood pressure, feeling of 'doom', and loss of consciousness. Some, but not necessarily all, of these symptoms are experienced. Acute management of anaphylaxis must be simple, swift and effective. Food anaphylaxis is a very serious life-threatening reaction requiring specialist medical attention.

Where to go for competent diagnosis and support

Your GP or hospital A&E should refer you to a paediatrician who has a special interest in allergies or to an allergy specialist.

Every effort must be made to identify the trigger of the reaction. You and your family will need education on how to avoid the food allergen (this should be provided by an experienced dietitian) and how to recognise further reactions. The specialist will devise an appropriate rescue treatment plan (see following page) for your child in the

Irish Food Allergy Network (IFAN)

The website of the Irish Food Allergy Network, www.ifan.ie, has a lot of very useful information on the incidence, diagnosis and management of food allergy.

quality of life

Children with severe food allergies are faced with food and social restrictions due to the potentially life-threatening nature of their condition. This inevitably affects their quality of life. In one study from the UK children with severe peanut allergy reported a poorer quality of life than children of the same age with diabetes. Clinical psychologists can provide invaluable help and support to children and their families trying to meet the day to day demands of living with severe food allergy. Hopefully in the future, as medical research advances, immune therapies, including vaccines, will become available so that children with allergies will be able to enjoy a normal diet without them or their parents having to worry about such stringent levels of food avoidance.

event of severe reaction, especially anaphylaxis, and it is a good idea to get a written copy of this plan. A child with severe food allergy should receive regular medical follow-up.

Steps to manage the risk of anaphylaxis

Fatal anaphylaxis is rare. Once you have received help and advice from your doctor, nurse and dietitian there will be many things you can do to reduce the risk of another episode of anaphylaxis and also to ensure that prompt and correct treatment is provided if a reaction does occur.

Most fatal and near fatal reactions happen when eating away from home. Your dietitian will advise you on eating out, reading food labels, hidden allergens etc. Children with severe food allergy should always wear some form of identification providing medic alert information. See page 196 for information on where to obtain identification products.

Rescue treatment plan

Even with allergen avoidance advice up to 50 per cent of families experience an accidental exposure within 12–18 months of diagnosis. If your child has or is at risk of a severe food allergy, your paediatrician/allergy specialist may prescribe an adrenaline auto-injector pen so that in an emergency you can give your child an adrenaline injection. Adrenaline works by restoring any loss in blood pressure and relaxing muscles. It will help reduce swelling and improve breathing. It will buy you time, allowing you to bring your child to the safety of emergency medical facilities.

a family matter
Food allergy is a whole family issue and it is essential that every single person involved in your child's care is educated about the allergy. You will also need to ensure that your child's school and friends' parents are fully informed.

The prospect of having to inject your child with adrenaline can be terrifying. But be reassured—your doctor and/or nurse will educate you on how to give adrenaline correctly. Trainer pens are available and these are a very useful teaching aid. Once you know how to give adrenaline correctly you will be able to save your child's life in the event of an anaphylactic reaction.

If an adrenaline auto-injector pen has been recommended, your doctor and/or nurse will provide you and your family with education and advice on:

- When to use an adrenaline auto injector
- How to use an adrenaline auto injector
- When to carry an adrenaline auto injector
- Storage/disposal of an adrenaline auto injector
- Expiry date of adrenaline auto injector

New Irish laws were signed by the Minister for Health in October 2015 allowing more life-saving rescue medicines including adrenaline auto injectors (AAIs) to be administed by trained members of the public in life-saving situations. These new laws allow organisations such as colleges, workplaces and sports venues to hold AAIs and arrange for staff to be trained in their use. Pharmacists are also able to supply and administer these medicines to individuals in emergency circumstances.

You must make sure that:
- Everyone knows what the child can eat and do.
- Friends and babysitters are aware of the risk of anaphylaxis.
- Your child's day care centre or school is aware of the risk of anaphylaxis.
- The day care centre or school is trained to administer adrenaline.
- The centre or school has 2 adrenaline auto injectors.
- Medic Alert information is to hand.

While it is important to plan for an emergency, this shouldn't overshadow the child or exclude them. Visit anaphylaxisireland.ie to download a free resource pack for schools, 'Managing Chronic Health Conditions at School'. This resource pack includes a section on managing anaphylaxis in school. The website also contains an excellent presentation from 2012 by Dr. Mary Keogan, Clinical Immunologist, Beaumont Hosptial, called '10 things we have learnt from our patients'.

Note If you have to give your child an adrenaline injection, always call an ambulance afterwards even if your child shows signs of improvement. A biphasic reaction can sometimes occur where symptoms go away at first but come back hours later. Therefore it's important to go to hospital and remain under observation for at least four hours.

Avoiding foods causing an allergic reaction

The only way to treat food allergy is to avoid the offending food, whether the allergy is IgE-mediated or non-IgE-mediated. How strictly a food needs to be avoided will depend on the severity and type of allergy. Your doctor will advise you accordingly. For example, in mild to moderate milk allergy, small traces of milk in cooked foods can be eaten without causing a reaction but milk, cream, cheese, yogurt and ice-cream should be avoided.

A breastfed baby with a cow's milk allergy can usually continue to breastfeed but the mother will need to exclude all sources of cow's milk from her diet.

While the potential of foods such as peanuts and seeds to cause an allergic reaction is not reduced by cooking, some egg-allergic children can eat well-cooked egg, for example in cake, but need to avoid raw or lightly cooked egg.

Removing foods from the diet

At first glance it may seem simple to remove a particular food from the diet. However, careful planning is needed to avoid such foods as milk, egg, peanut and wheat which are added to many different products. For example, hidden sources of milk include some brands of sausages and beef burgers, some crisps and Special K breakfast cereal.

Peanuts may be used as an ingredient in many different foods including cakes, biscuits, ice-cream, cereal bars, chocolate, salads, and sauces such as pesto and satay.

Substitutes for staple dietary foods such as milk and wheat will be needed to ensure the diet continues to provide all essential nutrients for the growing child or breastfeeding mother. A visit to the dietitian will provide you with all the necessary information. The book *Food Allergies: Enjoying Life with Severe Food Allergy* by Tanya Wright also provides a lot of really useful information.

Avoid nuts

Peanuts are not actually nuts—they are legumes. They are commonly called monkey nuts or ground nuts. Tree nuts are true nuts and include hazelnuts, brazil nuts, walnuts, cashew nuts and pecan nuts among others.

Children with peanut allergy may not be allergic to tree nuts and vice versa. However, up to 50% of children with peanut allergy will develop tree nut allergy. All peanut-allergic children should avoid tree nuts from first diagnosis until tested for tree nut sensitivity using a skin prick test or Specific IgE blood test. Negatively tested, tree nuts can be introduced to the home diet. This can help make the diet easier to follow but it is very important to continue to avoid tree nuts in prepared foods and out of home meals due to the risk of contamination and/or substitution by peanut.

Food labels

The greatest risk of triggering an allergic reaction lies in accidental exposure. Looking at food labels it is clear that this risk is enormous so label reading has to be the cornerstone of managing a food allergy.

Education is needed on how to read food labels and correctly identify the different names for common foods. A wallet sized laminated card giving the different ingredient names for a food can be a very useful aid when shopping.

By law all pre-packed foods must carry a list of ingredients. Current food labelling rules stipulate that every pre-packed food, including alcoholic drinks, sold in Ireland or anywhere in the EU must show clearly on the label if they contain any of the ingredients or their derivatives on the list on the next page.

Different names for milk in ingredients list	Different names for egg in ingredients list
Casein or curd	Egg yolk
Caseinates	Egg white
Hydrolysed casein	Egg protein
Whey, whey solids	Pasteurised egg
Whey protein	Frozen or dried egg
Whey sugar	Egg powder
Hydrolysed whey protein	Albumin
Lactose	Globulin
Skimmed milk powder	Lecithin E322 (can be soya or egg, more commonly soya)
Milk solids	Lysozyme
Non-fat milk solids	Ovalbumin or ovoglobulin or ovomucin or ovotransferrin or
Butter fat/Butter milk	ovovitellin
Ghee	Silici albuminate
Margarine	Vitellin
Lactoglobulin	
Cream/Artificial Cream	

ingredients that must be listed on pre-packed foods in the EU

- Celery
- Eggs
- Fish
- Mustard
- Peanuts
- Sesame seeds
- Soya beans
- Cereal containing gluten, including wheat, rye, barley, oats, khorasan, kamut and spelt. (It is important to note the word gluten may not actually appear on the label)
- Crustaceans—all species of crustaceans (e.g. lobster, crab, prawns, langoustines)
- Sulphites and sulphur dioxide (preservatives used in some foods and drinks) at levels above 10 parts per million
- Tree nuts such as almonds, hazelnuts, walnuts, Brazil nuts, cashews, pecan, pistachios and macadamia. Note: chestnuts and pinenuts are not included
- Milk (including lactose)
- Lupin
- Molluscs

The presence of any of the ingredients on the previous page, or their derivatives, must be emphasised on the food label list of ingredients through a typeset that clearly distinguishes them from the rest of the list of ingredients e.g. by means of the font, style or background colour.

Here are two examples of the types of ingredients listed on pre-packed products.

Ingredients listed on dessert yogurt label

Yogurt (**Milk**), Sugar, Water, Cocoa Butter, **Milk** Powder, Rice Flour, Cocoa Mass, Modified Starch, **Wheat** Flour (**Gluten**), Whey Powder (**Milk**) Flavourings, Lactose (**Milk**), Stabilisers: Carob Bean Gum, Guar Gum, Acacia Gum, **Barley** Malt, Salt, Colour: Carotenes, Emulsifier: **Soya** Lecithin
Allergy advice: see ingredients in **bold**.
May also contain Nut and/or Egg traces

Ingredients listed on biscuits label

Wheat flour, Sugar, Vegetable Fat (Palm), Glucose – Fructose Syrup, Maize Starch, Raising Agents (Ammonium Bicarbonate, Sodium Bicarbonate), **Milk** Powder, **Barley** Malt Extract, Salt, Emulsifier (**Soya** Lecithin), Flavours, Antioxidant (Sodium **Metabisulphite**).
For allergens, including cereals containing gluten, see ingredients in **bold**.
Produced in a factory handling Tree Nuts, Egg but on a different line.

other products to avoid

Children with severe food allergies may need to avoid any cosmetics, toiletries or perfumes containing natural extracts of foods. For information on the names of different ingredients used in these products visit www.ctpa.org.uk. Look under 'how are cosmetics regulated' followed by 'ingredient labelling'. Other items which may contain common food allergens include some medicines, pet food and washing up liquids.

These two lists of ingredients clearly state whether the food contains one of the 14 allergens listed under the labelling law. This is very useful when checking a food for the presence of an allergen. However, food labelling is in its infancy and mistakes have been made. It is a good idea always to read thoroughly through the list of ingredients. If you think a food has been labelled incorrectly you should report this to the Food Safety Authority of Ireland (Tel 01–817 1300 or info@fsai.ie).

Remember, too, that ingredients used in a food can change and for this reason you should read through the list of ingredients every single time you buy the food, even if it has been eaten only recently without problems. Also, the same product can contain different ingredients in different countries.

Be wary of foods making claims such as 'dairy free'. It is vital to read through the list of ingredients to verify a claim. Some 'non dairy' creamers or coffee whiteners and 'milk free' chocolate contain milk.

Non-prepacked foods

Since December 13th 2014, these 14 specific food allergens must also be declared on all non-prepacked foods including food and food items provided by restaurants, take-aways, pubs, food stalls, shops, supermarkets and childcare facilities. Allergens must be declared in writing and this information must be easily located and accessible to the consumer. Ideally the information should be presented in close proximity to the relevant food item e.g. written alongside the item on a menu or stored in a central location, such as a folder kept on the consumer side of the counter.

'May contain' warnings

We can see on the dessert yogurt ingredients list above a 'may contain' warning. This type of warning limits food choice for people with allergies even further.

While a food may not have a particular allergen, e.g. peanut or egg, as one of its ingredients, the manufacturer can't be sure that the product doesn't accidentally contain small amounts. Cross contamination may occur if different foods share the same production line or even if they are produced in the same factory.

'May contain' warnings are used extensively by the food industry and many people feel that these advisory warnings are sometimes given without good reason. However, for somebody with a severe food allergy, ignoring these warnings is akin to playing Russian roulette. The UK Food Standards Agency and a number of public interest groups are working to reduce the use of 'may contain' warnings. Indeed the Food Standards Agency has guidelines for food companies on how to determine whether or not allergen advisory labelling is appropriate.

Cross contamination

Children with severe food allergies can react to even trace amounts of the offending food allergen. For example, in ice-cream parlours, deli counters, sandwich and salad bars the same serving utensils are often used for different foods and a serving utensil may unintentionally become contaminated with a particular food allergen. This is known as cross contamination and in certain situations the risk of accidental exposure by this means can be high.

the MMR vaccine

The MMR vaccine can be safely given to children with egg allergy including those with severe allergy. This is because the MMR vaccine is grown on chick cells, not the egg white or yolk. All children with egg allergy, including those with severe allergy should receive the MMR vaccination in the normal manner at their GPs.

Food Allergen Alert Service

The Food Safety Authority of Ireland (FSAI) provides a free e-mail and SMS text service directly informing the consumer of the presence of allergens in inappropriately labelled foods e.g. missing or incorrect allergen labelling. You can subscribe to these alerts via the FSAI's website www.fsai.ie or telephone the advice line 1890 33 66 77

information on food labelling

can be obtained from the Food Safety Authority of Ireland advice line 1890 336677 or (01) 817 1300 or www.fsai.ie, info@fsai.ie or their UK counterpart Food Standards Agency www.food.gov.uk

Any of the following may be cross-contaminated:

- Chopping boards, knives and cooking utensils used during food preparation either in the home or in restaurants.
- Children's toys, including sand pits and paddling pools.
- Production lines of manufactured foods.
- Cooking oil used to fry different foods.

Cross reactions

As mentioned earlier, it is the protein in a food that triggers an allergic reaction from the immune system. Certain foods, especially if they belong to the same family, can contain proteins which are alike, e.g. sheep's, goat's and cow's milk all have similar proteins.

Where foods share very similar proteins there is a high risk of cross reactivity which means that the development of an allergy to one food can quickly be followed by allergies to the other foods. About 80 per cent of children allergic to cow's milk are also allergic to goat's milk.

Due to the high risk of cross reactivity sheep's, buffalo's or goat's milk should not be given to infants or children with a cow's milk allergy. Sometimes cross reactions can occur between food and non food stuffs that share a similar chemical structure. For example, it is common for people with a birch pollen allergy also to be allergic to celery.

'Free from' lists

Some supermarkets or food companies produce lists of their own-brand products free from specific food allergens. Many people find these invaluable. The one disadvantage to these lists is that they can quickly become out of date if, for example, a product is discontinued or its ingredients change. The company may not always contact you to alert you to an ingredient change and it is advisable to always read through the list of ingredients.

Precautions when eating out

The majority of allergic reactions occur outside the home. Convincing waiting staff that food allergies are real and getting accurate information about ingredients are just two of the problems encountered. Under the EU Food Information to Consumers (FIC) Regulation restaurants and take-aways are legally obliged to provide written food allergen information for all menu items including daily specials, sauces, condiments and beverages. The information can be placed alongside each written menu item or alternatively can be provided centrally in one or a number of conspicuous locations on

atopic diseases

Food allergy belongs to a group of diseases known as atopic diseases which includes asthma, eczema and hay fever. The incidence of atopic diseases has increased considerably over the past 30 years. In Europe an atopic disease affects about one quarter of all children.

the premises in hard copy or electronic format. Regardless of how the information is made available, it must be easily located, accessed and understood by the consumer. A child with a food allergy and his or her family should continue to enjoy eating out but some simple precautions will need to be taken.

- For children with peanut allergies it is best to avoid 'high risk' restaurants such as Chinese, Malaysian, Thai and Indian.
- Avoid self service restaurants, salad bars etc. as there is a high risk of cross contamination.
- Avoid fried foods such as chips if there is a risk of cross contamination of the cooking oil.
- Try to speak with the chef or restaurant manager in advance at a time when they are not very busy. It is always better to speak with the chef rather than a waiter or waitress.
- Keep food choices simple: avoid sauces, dressings, relishes, garnishes and dips.
- When giving an order ask for the food allergy to be written on it.
- It is important that the restaurant staff are fully aware of the seriousness of the allergy and if you are not confident of this, it is better to eat somewhere else
- Larger chain restaurants, with good ingredient information and static menus, can be a safer option.
- It may be a good idea to eat in the same restaurant regularly.
- If you have been prescribed rescue medications such as liquid anti-histamines and/or an adrenaline auto-injector pen by your doctor, ensure you always have your medications with you when eating out and are prepared to use them if necessary.

Going on holiday abroad

Careful planning is needed when taking a holiday abroad. Sometimes it can be necessary to bring your own food and it is always a good idea to obtain translation cards in the relevant language. Useful websites include: www.glutenfreepassport.com, www.allergylifestyle.com and www.yellowcross.co.uk.

Substitute foods

All children on an exclusion diet must be carefully assessed to ensure they have an adequate nutritional intake as excluding staple foods such as milk or wheat increases the risk of dietary deficiencies and malnutrition. Growing children are particularly vulnerable. For example, cow's milk is an important source of protein and calcium in the diet and several studies have demonstrated that the nutritional status of children on milk-free diets is less than ideal. Young children on a milk-free diet have been shown to be smaller and thinner than the national average. A study by Trinity College Dublin's school of medicine showed that even after calcium supplementation the average calcium intake of those avoiding milk was unacceptably low.

Dairy-free alternatives include a range of soya milks, yogurts and cheeses as well as ice-creams and chocolate spreads. Babies on a milk-free diet should take a suitable infant formula milk until at least 2 years of age or alternatively take a combined calcium and vitamin D supplement.

As discussed earlier, soya formula is no longer the first choice for infants with cow's milk protein allergy. Instead it is better to give a formula with confirmed reduced allergenicity such as Aptamil Pepti 1 or Nutramigen 1. Both of these formulas are cow's milk based but the protein has been broken down extensively into tiny fragments that cannot trigger an allergic reaction. They are classed as 'extensively hydrolysed' formulas. These formulas are available over the counter from pharmacies but if you buy them using a prescription their cost can be reclaimed under the drug payment scheme.

Hydrolysed formulas smell and taste very different to cow's milk infant formula and breast milk. Older babies, especially after 6 months of age, have a more well-developed sense of taste so may refuse at first to drink the hydrolysed formula but they usually adapt well to the taste. Sometimes it can help to dip the teat of the bottle in another milk substitute e.g. soya milk or expressed breast milk just before feeding. Your baby will smell this milk as the teat is placed in his or her mouth and may react better to the hydrolysed formula!

It may help also to add a very small amount of something with a sweet flavour, e.g. a drop of vanilla essence, to the hydrolysed formula to help improve the taste. If your baby accepts the formula, slowly reduce the amount of added flavouring until you are no longer adding any. Don't add any of these flavourings for more than a week to 10 days.

If you are breastfeeding your baby but are also giving an occasional bottle of formula, and you have a good milk supply it might help to mix a small amount of hydrolysed formula with expressed breast milk. Gradually increase the amount of hydrolysed formula mixed with breast milk and this will allow your baby, little by little, to get used to the taste of the formula.

It may not be possible to get some babies to accept the taste of hydrolysed formula; in this case, the best thing to do is give your baby a soya infant formula, provided your doctor is in agreement.

A very small number of babies with cow's milk allergy may be allergic to extensively hydrolysed formulas. In this case a formula made from synthetic amino acids will be needed, such as Neocate or Nutramigen Puramino. Follow-on formulas suitable from 6 months are also available—Aptamil Pepti 2 and Nutramigen 2.

Egg-free alternatives include egg-free mayonnaise and egg-free omelette and pancake mixes. Egg replacers are available from pharmacies and they can be used in baking e.g. egg white replacer can be used to make pavlova. Again, if you buy them using a prescription their cost can be reclaimed under the drug payment scheme.

Non-dairy and soya-free alternatives include rice milk, oat milk and almond milk. Rice milk should not be given to children under 4½ years of age, due to concerns about the presence of naturally occuring arsenic. When buying a non-dairy milk, always try to choose one that has been fortified with calcium of around 120mg per 100 ml. Soya- and dairy-free ice-creams are also available.

Gluten-free and/or wheat-free products are now available in many supermarkets which carry an extensive range including breads, crackers, pastas, pizza bases and biscuits. If your local supermarket does not carry a wide range of substitute foods, it can be a good idea to visit your local health food store. If you are unable to find a particular product it is always worth asking the shop if they can order it on your behalf. Alternatively it may be possible to order some substitute foods on line from e.g. www.goodnessdirect.co.uk.

Remember to be discerning when buying substitute foods, always check normal everyday foods first to see if they are suitable. It should only be necessary to buy specialist foods if there is no everyday equivalent available.

Prevention of food allergy in high-risk babies

Medical research has clearly shown that if a women smokes during pregnancy, or if other people are smoking nearby, her child has an increased risk of developing wheezy bronchitis and asthma. However, although a lot of research has been done in the area there is no such strong evidence to support dietary measures to prevent food allergy. There is evidence only to support prevention measures targeted at 'high risk' babies during the first year of life.

A high-risk baby is a baby whose mother or father or sibling is affected by an atopic disease such as asthma, eczema, hay fever or food allergy. Atopic diseases tend to run in families and family history is the strongest predictor of allergy. A child has a 20 per cent chance of developing an allergic disease if one parent has an atopic disease, and a 40 per cent chance if both parents have an atopic disease. Up to 50 per cent of children with food allergy have no family history of atopic disease. Measures for the prevention of food allergy should only be applied to high-risk infants. They are of no benefit to low-risk infants.

If you are pregnant or have just had a new baby, and you or your partner or one of your children suffers from asthma, eczema, food allergy or hay fever your baby falls into the high-risk category and you should follow the current recommendations (see following pages) for preventing the development of a food allergy. Unfortunately, the present level of medical knowledge falls short of providing all the answers on how best to feed high-risk infants. It is likely that allergy prevention recommendations will be updated in time as new evidence becomes available.

Frequently asked questions

What foods should be avoided during pregnancy and while breastfeeding?

No foods need to be avoided during pregnancy or while breast feeding. Women were previously advised that they may wish to avoid eating peanuts during pregnancy or while breast feeding if there was a positive family history of allergy. However the latest research now shows that eating or not eating peanuts seems to have no effect on the chances of your baby developing a peanut allergy.

What is the best feed for my baby?

Exclusive breastfeeding for the first 4 – 6 months of life, irrespective of the baby's risk of allergy, is recommended. It is also the most effective dietary measure for the prevention of allergic diseases and gives the best start in life.

In terms of allergy prevention breast milk has a number of components that have a positive effect on the baby's developing immune system and enhance their natural defences. However, exclusive breastfeeding does not guarantee that your baby will never develop an allergy.

What formula should I give my baby if I am unable or choose not to breastfeed or need to give a supplement to the breastfeeds?

In the past mothers may have been advised to offer their baby a partially hydrolysed formula such as SMA H.A. Infant Milk or an extensively hydrolysed formula such as Aptamil Pepti 1 or Nutramigen 1. Following an extensive review of the research in this area, the UK Committe of Toxicity on Chemicals in Food, Consumer Products and the Environment (COT) issued a statement in February 2016 advising that there is no evidence to suggest giving these formula will help prevent food allergy or autoimmune diseases such as Type 1 Diabetes. Where breast milk is not available, routine cow's milk based infant formula should be given. The World Allergy Organisation recommends prebiotics for non exclusively breastfed infants. Aptamil, Cow & Gate and SMA infant formulas all contain prebiotics. For more information on prebiotics please see Chapter 4 page 46–7.

Is it all right to give my baby soya or goat's milk formula instead of a formula with reduced allergencity?

No. Goat's milk or soya infant formulas are not recommended. They should not be given instead of a formula with reduced allergenicity. Goat's milk protein is very similar to cow's milk protein and a cross reaction could occur.

When should I wean my baby and what foods should I give?

There is a natural window of opportunity from 4-6 months of age (inclusive) in which babies are capable of tolerating potentially allergenic foods. Eating food allergens during this time promotes life long tolerance. Unnecessary avoidance promotes long term allergy.

It is important not to introduce solids before 4 months (17 weeks) of age. However, there is no advantage to delaying weaning past 6 months of age and indeed this will be harmful to the baby's development. (See Chapter 6.)

Young babies' guts are immature and can be 'leaky' allowing food proteins to pass from the gut into the blood stream. Over time the gut matures. Early exposure, i.e. before 17 weeks, to certain foods appears to be an important factor in the development of allergy, so it's best to start weaning with low-allergenic foods. These include baby rice, puréed root vegetable (carrot, turnip, parsnip), puréed fruit (banana, apple, pear).

Whole nuts are unsuitable for children under 5 years because of choking risk. While nut products are suitable from 6 months of age for low-risk infants, opinions differ on when nut products should be introduced for high-risk infants. Read about 'The LEAP Study' below.

High-allergenic foods/food groups should be introduced one at a time with a gap of 3 days between each new food/food group. There is no benefit to delaying the introduction of high allergenic foods.

The milk or dairy food group includes cow's milk, yogurt and cheese and the wheat food group includes bread, pasta and cereal. To check for a potential food allergy only one food from a food group needs to be eaten. Sometimes a food can contain more than one ingredient and it may be best to add these foods to the diet one at a time to allow detection of reactions for individual components.

It can be a good idea to keep a food symptom diary during this period as it may prove useful in identifying allergic symptoms. By the age of 12 months all the major allergenic foods which would normally be suitable for a child of this age should have been introduced.

The LEAP Study

In March 2015 results from the LEAP (Learning Early about Peanut Allergy) Study were published in the New England Journal of Medicine (a copy of the paper is available on the Irish Food Allergy Network website, www.ifan.ie). The LEAP study showed that children at risk of food allergies can be prevented from developing a peanut allergy by including peanuts in their diet from around 6 months of age. Children with severe eczema or egg allergy or both are known to be at risk of peanut allergy. 640 infants aged between 4–11 months of age with severe eczema, egg allergy, or both, participated in the study.

Results from the study showed that the risk of peanut allergy can be reduced by up to 80% by including peanuts in infant diets.

If your child is at risk of peanut allergy it is essential that they have a skin prick test to check for sensitization to peanuts prior to introducing peanut into their diet. 85% of peanut allergic children react on their first exposure to peanut. Therefore to ensure peanut is introduced safely it should only be included in the diet following a skin prick test and in consultation with your doctor. Contact details for doctors specialising in food allergy are available at the end of this chapter.

How long should I continue to breastfeed?

Exclusive breastfeeding for the first 6 months of life gives maximum benefit to the baby. Breast milk or infant formula milk is required for all babies until their first birthday as normal cow's milk is not a suitable drink before this time.

Babies who are exclusively breastfed can be given a cow's milk based formula from 4 to 6 months onwards if being weaned or supplementary feeds are required. The cow's milk-based formula should be treated in the same way as a high-allergenic food. It may be best to start off with a small volume initially and not to introduce any other high-allergenic foods for 3 days following the introduction of the cow's milk-based infant formula.

What about eczema and allergy prevention?

New research is showing that management of eczema is important in preventing food allergy. The skin acts as a barrier. If the skin is broken down food proteins can enter the body this way and trigger a reaction from the immune system. For babies with eczema a good skin care routine is essential in order to optimise skin barrier function. It is very important to stop any inflammation in the skin and if your doctor has prescribed a mild steroidal cream such as 1% hydrocortisone, be sure to use it. The cheeks are a particularly weak point in the skin in babies up until one year of age. If eczema is present on the cheeks, your doctor may advise you to apply vaseline to the affected skin to help create a barrier.

Further information

Doctors specialising in the diagnosis and management of allergy

You will need a referral letter from your GP.

Dublin: Dr. Aideen Byrne, Paediatric Allergist, AMNCH, Tallaght Tel 01 4142000 and Our Lady's Children's Hospital Crumlin, Tel 01 4096013 or e-mail: allergy.secretary@olchc.ie

Cork: Prof. Jonathan Hourihane, Head of Paediatrics and Child Health, Clinical Investigations Unit, Cork University Hospital, Cork, Tel 021 4901237

Antrim: Dr Trevor Brown, Consultant Paediatrician, Children's Allergy Service. The Ulster Hospital, Dundonald, Belfast, BT16 IRH, Tel 028 9048 4511

Galway: Dr. Edina Moylett, Consultant Paediatrician, University College Hospital Galway, Tel 091 524222

Louth: Dr. John Fitzsimons, Paediatric Allergist, Our Lady of Lourdes Hospital, Drogheda, Tel 041 9837601

Midlands: Dr. Imelda Lambert, Consultant Paediatrician, Mullingar Regional Hospital, Tel 044 9340221

& Dr. Paul Gallagher, Consultant Paediatrician, Portlaoise Hospital, Tel 057 8621364

Other doctors who may be able to provide allergy testing include: consultant dermatologists for children with eczema; consultant respiratory physicians for children with asthma; consultant paediatricians with a special interest in allergy—contact details should be available from your GP or local hospital; clinical immunologists work in a number of adult hospitals and may accept referrals for children with suspected allergies—contact details should be available from either your GP or hospital.

Dietitians in private practice
If you attend a doctor at a public hospital, he or she will be able to refer you to a dietitian. A hospital dietitian always needs a written referral (from a doctor working in the hospital) before he or she can see a patient. If you would like to see a dietitian, let your doctor know and a referral can be made. If you attend a private allergy specialist, a referral to the dietitian can also be made. You will need to pay an additional consultation fee to the dietitian.

   Alternatively, to find a dietitian working in private practice in your area, contact the Irish Nutrition and Dietetic Institute, the professional body for dietitians working in Ireland, Tel 01–280 4839, info@indi.ie, www.indi.ie. The honorary secretary of the Irish Food Allergy Network (IFAN) Ruth Charles, Paediatric Dietitan sees patients privately, info@nutrikids.ie, www.nutrikids.ie

Further information
A–Z directory of allergens is listed on the web page www.allallergy.net. Over 200 allergens are listed.

Action Against Allergy is a support charity providing information including holiday and accommodation, suppliers' lists, and newsletter. PO Box 278, Twickenham, TW1 4QQ, UK. Tel 0044 208 8922711, actionagainstallergy@btconnect.com, www.actionagainstallergy.co.uk

Allergen Alert Cards these are credit-card style cards and are available to buy from the website www.dietarycard.co.uk

Allergy UK is a national medical charity providing up to date information on all aspects of allergy. Planwell House, LEFA Business Park, Edgington Way, Sidcup, Kent, DA14 5BH. Helpline: 0044 1322 619898, info@allergyuk.org, www.allergyuk.org

Anaphylaxis Campaign (UK), 1 Alexandra Road, Farnborough, Hampshire GU14 6BU, UK. Helpline: 0044 1252 542029, info@anaphylaxis.org.uk, www.anaphylaxis.org.uk

Anaphylaxis Ireland www.anaphylaxisireland.ie

Cosmetics For information on the names of different ingredients in cosmetics, toiletries and perfumes see www.ctpa.org.uk, look under 'how are cosmetics regulated' followed by 'ingredient labelling'

Food Allergies: Enjoying Life with a Severe Food Allergy by Tanya Wright (ISBN 1-85959-039-X) is a very helpful book on food allergy

Labels The following websites give very useful information on food labels
Food Safety Authority of Ireland (FSAI), Tel 1890 33 66 77, www.fsai.ie, info@fsai.ie or
Food Standards Agency (FSA) www.food.gov.uk

Allergy Lifestyle is an Irish-owned company providing a wide range of products and information resources to help make life a little easier and safer for people living with food allergy. Products available from the online shop include an excellent range of identification 'jewllery' and wrist bands, personalised food allergy labels and translation cards in several languages for nut, dairy and egg allergies. Allergy Lifestyle, Innovation Hubs, GMIT Mayo, Castlebar, Co. Mayo. Tel 091 442377 / 0203 2873771, customercare@ allergylifestyle.com, www.allergylifestyle.com

Medic-Alert Foundation provides a selection of identification 'jewellery' with an internationally recognised medical symbol and 24 hour emergency telephone number for people with hidden medical conditions. MedicAlert House, 327-329 Witan Court, Upper Fourth Street, Milton Keynes, MK9 1EH, United Kingdom, Tel 0044 1908 951045, info@ medicalert.org.uk, www.medicalert.org.uk

Vegetarian and vegan diets for children

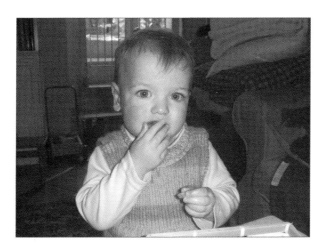

Following a vegetarian diet can have health benefits but only if the diet is carefully planned to include all the necessary nutrients. This is especially important for babies and young children. Parents who are committed to a vegan diet for their children have to take even more care to make sure that their nutritional needs are met. In fact, vegan diets are not recommended for young children as it is extremely difficult to ensure they receive all the essential nutrients for growth and development.

In this chapter we identify the areas that require special attention when following a vegetarian or vegan diet and advise how best to ensure that your child receives all the nutrients needed to thrive.

For our purposes we consider a vegetarian someone who does not eat meat, fish or poultry but does eat eggs and dairy products. Vegans exclude eggs and dairy products from their diet as well as meat, fish and poultry.

Most of this chapter applies to both vegetarian and vegan diets; where there are exceptions we indicate this.

vegetarian diets can be beneficial

According to the American Dietetic Association and Dietitians of Canada 'appropriately planned vegetarian diets are healthful, nutritionally adequate and provide health benefits in the prevention and treatment of certain diseases'. The diseases are obesity, cardiovascular disease, high blood pressure, diabetes and certain cancers.

Note the words 'appropriately planned': suitable replacement foods must be eaten instead of meat etc.

Iron

Iron is an essential nutrient that the body cannot manufacture itself; it therefore has to be included in the diet. Children, particularly toddlers, are very susceptible to iron-deficiency anaemia. A baby's iron stores received from the mother are depleted by the age of 6 months therefore it is important to provide good iron sources from 6 months onwards. When meat, which is an excellent source of iron, is excluded from a child's diet, parents need to make an extra effort to ensure the child is getting enough iron.

If your baby is taking formula milk, it may be useful to change to a follow-on formula at 6 months old as these formulas generally contain more iron than first and second formulas. Follow-on formulas also contain more calcium and protein.

Good sources of iron for vegetarians and vegans.

- Lentils, peas and beans, including baked beans—simple to prepare and very nutritious.
- Dark green, leafy vegetables e.g. spinach, cabbage, broccoli.
- Fortified cereals; one serving of breakfast cereal can contain up to

4 mg of iron. See page 200 for how that measures up to your child's daily needs. Read the labels of different brands and pick one that has iron added.

- Whole meal bread: 1 slice contains 1 mg of iron.
- Dried fruit—figs, apricots, raisins, currants, sultanas and dates—can be sprinkled on cereal or given as a healthy snack.
- Tofu.

For vegetarians only:

- Eggs—the iron is in the yolk so try to make sure your child eats that part at least.

Iron absorption: haem- and non-haem iron

The iron in red meat is known as 'haem-iron'. It is absorbed up to seven times more easily than the iron in cereals, vegetables and fruits which is known as 'non-haem iron'. Vegetarians and vegans therefore get all their iron as 'non-haem' iron. In addition, certain substances further interfere with iron absorption. These include phytates, tea, coffee, oxalates, cocoa and some spices.

Phytates are substances made of the mineral phosphorous; they are found in cereal grains, peas, beans, lentils and nuts. They attach themselves to minerals such as iron, calcium, and zinc and interfere with their absorption in the body. This is unfortunate considering a lot of foods that contain phytates are sources of iron for vegetarians and vegans. However, some food preparation techniques such as soaking beans and leavening breads can help to reduce the effects of the phytates.

Vitamin C can also counteract some of the effects of phytates and help the body to absorb iron from non-meat sources. It is contained in citrus fruits, berries and certain vegetables. The vitamin C in a glass of orange juice taken in the morning with iron-fortified cereal converts the iron in the cereal into a form that is easier for the body to absorb.

It is recommended that children aged 1–3 years take 8mg iron a day and children aged 4–6 years take 9mg iron a day.

Some studies have shown that vegetarians and vegans may need to eat almost twice the recommended amount of iron for their age due to the fact that the non-haem iron is harder to absorb. This can be difficult to achieve but you can try to ensure that your child takes iron-rich foods every day (aim for about 3 portions a day) and follow the advice below about testing your child for anaemia.

vegan diets are not recommended for young children.

In January 2008 the European Society for Paediatric Gastroentorology, Hepatology and Nutrition (ESPGHAN) stated that infants on a vegan or macro-biotic diet with limited or no animal foods have a high risk of developing nutritional deficiencies. They concluded that 'infants and young children should not receive a vegan diet.'

advice from dietitians

Parents who are committed to a vegan diet for their children need to take special care to ensure that their nutritional needs are met and should seek advice from a qualified dietitian. Visit www.indi.ie to find a qualified, properly trained dietitian in your area. There may be a dietitian attached to your local health centre.

On the other hand, your child's iron level may be high enough even without consuming the recommended value as the need for iron varies from person to person according to different factors. There is also some evidence to suggest that vegetarians and vegans become better at absorbing iron over time as their bodies adapt to a lower iron intake.

Recommendations for iron intake
- Children aged 1–3 years need 8 mg iron a day
- Children aged 4–6 years need 9 mg of iron a day

The table below lists the amount of iron contained in various foods. It will help you to estimate if your child is getting sufficient iron.

iron content in various foods suitable for vegetarians and vegans		
Food	Portion size	Iron (mg)
Special K	2 tablespoons (20 g)	2.3
Weetabix	1 biscuit	2.5
Ready Brek	2 tablespoons (20 g)	2.3
Cheerios	2 tablespoons (20 g)	2.3
Whole meal bread	1 slice (35 g)	1.0
Baked beans	half a small tin (100 g)	1.5
Tofu, firm	60 g	2.0
Kidney beans, cooked	2 heaped tablespoons (80 g)	1.7
Lentils, cooked	2 tablespoons	2.8
1 portion cooked spinach	2 tablespoons (80 g)	1.3
Raisins	1 tablespoon	1.0
Hummus	1 tablespoon (30 g)	0.6
Tahini	1 heaped teaspoon	2.0

Testing a child for anaemia

A child who is not getting enough iron will eventually become anaemic. However, anaemia can be difficult to identify. If your child is vegetarian or vegan you should arrange to have a full blood count done by your GP before the child's second birthday. The test will confirm whether your child is anaemic or not.

If your child's full blood count shows evidence of anaemia your GP will prescribe an iron supplement. Remember that iron supplements may cause your child's stools to darken. They can also cause constipation.

vitamin C and iron absorption

Don't forget to give a drink or food containing vitamin C at mealtimes to help with iron absorption.

Do not give your child an iron-only supplement without your doctor's advice and getting a full blood count done. Too much iron in the body can be dangerous. Some multivitamin and mineral tablets contain iron. However, such tablets are designed to supplement the diet—not to treat iron-deficiency anaemia.

You can also ask your GP to check your child's ferritin (store of iron) level to see if it is adequate. Generally the ferritin level drops before anaemia actually sets in.

If the first full blood count shows no anaemia another test may not be needed for a year or two. On the other hand if your child is anaemic more frequent tests will be needed.

sample meals to maximise iron intake on vegetarian and vegan diets

Breakfast
- Iron-fortified cereal with milk/soya milk and a handful of raisins scattered on the cereal

Vegetarian only
- Scrambled eggs on toast
- Boiled egg with toast 'soldiers'

Don't forget your glass of orange juice to help absorb the iron!

Lunch
- Baked beans on wholemeal toast
- Hummus in pitta bread pouches
- Lentil soup with a soft breadroll
- Minestrone soup containing pasta and beans
- Pasta salad with kidney beans and red peppers (red peppers contain vitamin C)

Vegetarian only
- Egg salad sandwich

Dinner
- Vegetarian bean chilli
- Vegetable and lentil curry
- Vegetable and tofu stir-fry
- Falafel in pitta bread

Vegetarian only
- Quiche
- Omelette or frittata
- Pizza Fiorentina (toppings include spinach and egg)
- Spaghetti Carbonara using asparagus instead of bacon

anaemia

A lack of iron in the diet is one of the main causes for concern for a child on a vegetarian or vegan diet. It can cause anaemia, a condition where the red blood cells are deficient in haemo-globin (which contains iron). Red blood cells carry oxygen around the body. This is why anaemic people may feel tired—because the body isn't getting enough oxygen. Anaemia in children can also affect their brain develop-ment. It is absolutely essential to make sure your child is getting enough iron every day.

an egg a day is ok

In the past we were told not to eat more than two eggs a week. However, as our knowledge of nutrition increases, we now know that it is fine to eat as many as seven eggs a week.

Omega-3 and omega-6 oils

Omega-3 and omega-6 oils are polyunsaturated fats. Linoleic acid (an omega-6 fat) and alphalinoleic acid (an omega-3 fat) are essential fats. 'Essential' means that the body is not able to make them so they must be included in the diet.

Omega-3 Vegetarians and vegans can get omega-3 oil from vegetable sources like walnut oil, rapeseed oil, linseed oil and flaxseed oil. Omega-3 oil from these sources is called 'alpha-linoleic acid' (ALA) which, in order to be of benefit, has to be converted by the body into EPA (eicosapentaenoic acid) and DHA (docosahexaenoic acid). It is not yet clear how easy it is for the body to convert ALA into EPA and DHA. One teaspoon of walnut oil or flaxseed oil would provide enough omega-3 for your child in one day if it was all converted into EPA and DHA, but as we have seen, it is not clear just how much the body converts. The oil can be taken directly or added into a salad dressing as these oils should not be heated. It is quite safe to eat more than one teaspoon of these oils a day.

Eggs, milk and orange juice fortified with omega-3 are now available but are not always suitable for vegetarians and vegans as sometimes the omega-3 oil is taken from an animal source.

Omega-6 is also called 'linoleic acid'. Most people eat quite a lot of omega-6 as it is in many foods, for example, lean meat, eggs and vegetable oils such as sunflower oil and corn oil. However, eating a lot of omega-6 fats can prevent the body from converting omega-3 fats into EPA and DHA. So it is important to eat a good balance of omega-3 and omega-6 oils. This is particularly important for people on diets excluding fish which is a direct source of EPA and DHA.

Oil in supplements Flaxseed oil is available as a supplement. DHA from sea-algae is available as a supplement in non-gelatin capsules. These are particularly useful for pregnant or breastfeeding mothers when a good intake is essential. They are generally available in health food shops.

Omega-3 and omega-6 sources for vegetarians and vegans
- Omega-3: walnut oil, rapeseed oil, linseed oil and flaxseed oil.
  Some food products fortified with omega-3 are suitable for vegans and vegetarians
- Omega-6: sunflower oil, corn oil, safflower oil and (for vegetarians only) eggs

olive oil contains mono-unsaturated fat and does not affect the conversion of Omega-3 oils to EPA and DHA. To prevent excessive intake of omega-6, use olive oil in addition to other oils.

DHA in breast milk

There is increasing evidence that long chain polyunsaturated fatty acids (LCPs), are important for brain and eye development in infants. Two LCPs are particularly relevant to growing infants: arachidonic acid (AA) and docosahexaenoic acid (DHA). There is some evidence that breast milk of vegetarian and vegan mothers can have lower levels of DHA compared to that of fish-eating mothers.

In order to provide enough DHA in breast milk it is advised that vegetarian and vegan breastfeeding women avoid excessive use of omega-6 oils and use more omega-3 oils.

This is because eating too much omega-6 oils can prevent the body converting omega-3 oils into DHA.

There are also supplements available in health food shops that contain DHA taken from sea-algae. These supplements are designed for vegetarians and vegans and can provide pregnant and breastfeeding mothers with a good source of DHA.

Vitamin B_{12}

Vitamin B_{12} performs a number of functions in the body. Deficiency causes pernicious anaemia. If left untreated this can sometimes result in irreversible damage to the nervous system. Most vegans and vegetarians have a high intake of folic acid which can mask the early signs of a vitamin B_{12} deficiency and can result in it remaining undiagnosed until neurological symptoms occur.

Breastfeeding and Vitamin B_{12}

If you are breastfeeding and not consuming enough vitamin B_{12} it will affect your baby's stores of vitamin B_{12} and they may become deficient. Infants breastfed by vegan mothers are particularly at risk of vitamin B_{12} deficiency. This can be very serious, causing permanent neurological damage and even death. A number of such cases of vitamin B_{12} deficiency have been documented in babies breastfed by vegan mothers who did not take a B_{12} supplement themselves or supplement their babies.

It is therefore essential that breastfeeding vegan and vegetarian mothers ensure that they are getting adequate amounts of vitamin B_{12} in their diet (about 1.9 micrograms a day) so that their babies do not become vitamin B_{12} deficient. Vitamin B_{12} is only found in foods of animal origin. However, that includes dairy products and eggs, so vegetarian breastfeeding mothers generally don't need to take a vitamin B_{12} supplement if they are consuming these foods regularly.

Vegan breastfeeding mothers do need to take a supplement or supplement their babies as the only sources of vitamin B_{12} for vegans are fortified milk substitutes, stocks, breakfast cereals and other fortified foods. It may be safer to supplement your baby directly to be absolutely sure he or she is getting all the vitamin B_{12} needed. See next page for suitable supplements containing vitamin B_{12}.

Vegan women also need to ensure they have a good intake of vitamin B_{12} during pregnancy.

vitamin B_{12} supplements for babies breastfed by vegan mothers

Ketovite liquid is one of the only vitamin supplements suitable for babies containing vitamin B_{12} and vitamin D. It can be given from one month onwards. The liquid does not contain vitamin B_2 (riboflavin) but Ketovite tablets contain vitamin B_2 as well as vitamin B_1, vitamin C, folic acid, vitamin E and other vitamins. These tablets can be crushed and given to infants in the liquid. A dose of 2.5 ml liquid and 1 tablet from 1 month of age will provide enough vitamin B_{12}, vitamin D and vitamin B_2 for your baby. Once your baby is 12 months old the dose of Ketovite liquid can be increased to 5 ml a day.

As always, it is best to obtain advice from your GP before giving your baby these supplements. Ketovite supplement is available on prescription only.

Bottle-feeding and Vitamin B$_{12}$

Both regular and soya infant formula contain vitamin B$_{12}$ so if your baby is drinking more than 500 ml of formula you do not need to give him or her a vitamin B$_{12}$ supplement unless otherwise advised by your GP. However, once your baby is weaned onto solids it is important to provide foods containing vitamin B$_{12}$.

soya formula for vegan babies

Soya formula is made to EU standards and contains all the nutrients a healthy baby needs to grow and develop normally. Regular soya milk is completely unsuitable for babies and should not be given as a main drink under the age of 24 months.

Soya formulas contain glucose syrup to provide carbohydrate for energy. It is completely safe for babies and is a necessary addition to soya formula. However, it is important to practice good dental hygiene if your child is drinking soya formula. Don't allow your child to take a bottle to bed as this can result in dental damage if teeth are effectively 'bathed' in formula all night. Introducing your baby to a feeding cup from the age of 6 months onwards and moving away from the bottle will help to prevent tooth decay.

Absorption of vitamin B$_{12}$

Recommended intakes of vitamin B$_{12}$ are usually based on the assumption that about 50 per cent of the vitamin B$_{12}$ eaten will be absorbed. Absorption is better if small amounts of vitamin B$_{12}$ fortified foods are taken regularly throughout the day rather than in one large dose. So if your child is not taking supplements he or she should take 3 servings of fortified food each containing about 1 microgram of vitamin B$_{12}$ spread out over the day with a few hours in between.

Vitamin B$_{12}$ supplements for vegan toddlers

If your child is eating enough vitamin B$_{12}$ from fortified foods a supplement may not be necessary.

However, considering a vegan diet is so limited, it is probably a good idea to continue supplementing your child with Ketovite or VEG 1 (see box) until the age of 5.

For vegetarians, Abidec Multivitamin drops could be continued up to the age of 5, at a dose of 0.3 ml twice daily, but if your child is eating a varied diet a supplement may not be needed.

There are no Irish recommendations relating to vitamin supplements for children over the age of 12 months.

Testing blood levels of vitamin B_{12}

If you are not giving supplements it may be advisable to get your child's B_{12} levels checked. Unfortunately, a simple blood vitamin B_{12} level is often not accurate for vegans as it can be affected by eating algaes or other plant foods that contain similar chemicals to vitamin B_{12}. Therefore, your doctor may have to request a test for something called methylmalonic acid (MMA). A raised level of MMA may suggest a deficiency of Vitamin B_{12}.

What to look for in supplements

When looking for a multivitamin and mineral supplement for your vegan child, look for one that contains vitamin B_{12}, vitamin B_2 and vitamin D, and ideally also iron and iodine.

VEG 1, available from the UK Vegan Society, contains vitamin B_{12}, vitamin B_2, vitamin B_6, vitamin D, folic acid, iodine and selenium. It is suitable from age one right up to adulthood. It can be bought online (www.vegansociety.com) and posted to customers in Ireland at a cost of £5.98 plus p & p.

children's daily vitamin B_{12} requirements

Age	Vitamin B_{12} (micrograms)
0–3 months	0.3
4–6 months	0.3
7–9 months	0.4
10–12 months	0.4
1–3 years	0.7
4–6 years	0.9

Vitamin B_{12} content of various foods

Vegetarian only	Vitamin B_{12} (micrograms)
1 glass unfortified cow's milk	1.8
1 egg	0.7
28g of cheddar cheese	0.7
1 average pot of natural yogurt	0.25
Vegetarian and vegan	
1 child's portion of Marmite	0.3
1 average bowl of fortified cereal	0.5
1 adult portion of Marmite	0.6

useful sources of vitamin B_{12}

Some products are marketed for vegans with claims that they contain vitamin B_{12} such as seaweeds, algaes, barley grass and many others but these are not adequate sources of vitamin B_{12} and it is not advisable to use them. The only useful sources of vitamin B_{12} for vegans are forti-fied foods (foods that have vitamin B_{12} added to them such as breakfast cereals, stocks and soya milks) and vitamin supplements.

stocks and yeast extracts

These can be a very useful addition to the diet of vegetarian and vegan children as they are generally high in vitamins and minerals. The following brands are available in Ireland.

- Vecon concentrated vegetable stock is available in health food stores. It contains vitamins A, B_1, B_2, Niacin, B_{12}, C and iron.
- Marmite yeast extract contains Vitamins B_1, B_2, niacin, folic acid and vitamin B_{12}. One 2 g child's serving size of Marmite provides 0.3 micrograms of vitamin B_{12}.
- Meridian foods make a yeast extract rich in vitamin B_{12}, available in health food shops.
- Marigold yeast flakes are also available in health food shops and contain vitamins B_1, B_2, B_6, (no B_{12}) folic acid and iron.

Note: Stocks and yeast extracts are high in salt so it is best to avoid giving them to children under one year old.

breastfeeding on vegetarian and vegan diets

Breast milk gives the best start for all babies and vegetarian and vegan babies are no exception. However, there are a few key nutrients that breastfeeding mothers on vegetarian and vegan diets need to be aware of especially vitamin B_{12} and vitamin D. Having a good intake of vitamin B_2 (riboflavin) and calcium is also very important for breastfeeding mothers.

Vitamin D

Vitamin D is very important for bone health as it plays a key role in calcium metabolism and bone formation. Before birth the baby builds up stores of vitamin D from the mother. This depends on the mother having good stores of vitamin D herself during her pregnancy.

Mature breast milk contains very little vitamin D and if a mother has poor stores of the vitamin the baby will get very little of it.

Breastfeeding mothers need to have some exposure to sunlight so that the skin can manufacture vitamin D (about 15 minutes a day without sunscreen with the face and hands exposed to the sun). However, in Ireland, because of limited sunlight, particularly during winter months, there is a high risk of developing vitamin D deficiency and of breast milk containing lower levels of vitamin D.

vitamin D is not naturally present in many foods. It is, however, present in eggs, fortified cereals, spreads, milks and other fortified foods. A deficiency of vitamin D in your baby's diet could cause rickets which is a condition where the bones are too soft and bend, causing bone deformities. Breastfed babies can be at risk of vitamin D deficiency so they need to be given a vitamin supplement.

Vitamin D supplements for breastfed babies

The Food Safety Authority of Ireland (FSAI) recommends that all exclusively and partially breastfed babies (taking less than 500ml formula per day) receive a vitamin D supplement from birth. A daily dose of 0.3 ml of Abidec Multivitamin drops for babies and children provides the recommended daily 5 micrograms of vitamin D.

After the first month, the babies of vegan mothers can be given Ketovite (liquid and tablet) instead of Abidec Multiviatamin drops. Abidec Multiviatamin drops contains vitamins A, B_1, B_2, B_6, C and D but not vitamin B_{12}. Breastfed babies of vegan and vegetarian mothers can continue on their vitamin supplements for the first year or until they are taking 500 ml of formula a day.

Sources of vitamin B_2 (riboflavin) for vegans

Riboflavin's role in the body is to help chemical reactions involved in metabolism of fats and glucose to take place . Milk and its products are the main dietary sources of riboflavin. Deficiency is rare in the general population but some studies have shown vegans to have lower intakes of riboflavin.

Sources of B_2 for vegans include fortified cereals, ground almonds, fortified milk substitutes, mushrooms, asparagus, broccoli, tahini, tofu, lentils, peas and seeds.

Breastfeeding mothers need to be particularly vigilant about regularly eating sources of vitamin B_2 or to supplement their intake.

Abidec Multivitamin drops contains vitamin B_2 as do Ketovite tablets and VEG 1.

> **tofu,** also known as 'bean curd' is made from fermented soy milk. It is often used in Asian cooking and is a good source of protein and iron. Tofu that has been set in calcium sulphate is an excellent source of calcium. You can get both firm and soft varieties of tofu and it can be fried, deep-fried, steamed, stuffed and served in many other ways.

Iodine and vegan diets

Most people receive iodine from milk so vegans are at a particular risk of iodine-deficiency. In adults, iodine deficiency causes hypothyroidism. If a woman has a severely restricted intake of iodine during pregnancy her baby can be born with severe developmental delay and even deafness. Pregnant women need about 130 micrograms of iodine per day.

> **seaweed** is an excellent source of iodine and should be included in the vegan diet for this reason.

A study done on 54 Irish-born pregnant women attending the National Maternity Hospital, Dublin, in 2004/5 found that up to 55 per cent of the women in the study displayed evidence of dietary iodine deficiency.

Breastfeeding mothers need about 160 micrograms a day. If you are breastfeeding and consuming adequate iodine yourself, your breast milk should contain adequate iodine. Formula provides iodine to bottle-fed babies.

Seaweed and iodised salt are good sources of iodine for vegans. Seaweed-based products are available in most health food shops. Cerebos Extra Fine Iodised Table Salt is one brand of iodised table salt available in Ireland and can be bought in most supermarkets. It contains 1150 micrograms iodine per 100 g salt.

Remember that salt should not be added to your baby's diet at less than one year old. Some vegan supplements such as VEG 1, available on the UK vegan website, contain iodine.

Don't take in more than the recommended amount of iodine by over-consuming seaweeds and iodised salt.

children's iodine needs

Food safety Authority of Ireland recommendations

Age	Micrograms per day
0–3 months	50
4–6 months	60
7–9 months	60
10–12 months	60
1–3 years	70
4–6 years	90

feeding babies on vegetarian or vegan diets

Vegetarian babies can be moved onto cow's milk at the age of 12 months if their diet is varied and they are getting adequate iron. However, you may prefer to breast-feed for longer. If you are concerned about the quality of your baby's diet, it is best to continue with breast milk or formula until the age of 2 years.

Vegan babies should be breast fed or given formula until they are 2 years old; this will provide extra protein, vitamins and minerals.

Vitamin A for vegans

Vitamin A helps maintain the health of skin, strengthens immunity from infections and is essential for vision. Non-vegans can get vitamin A (retinol) directly from foods of animal origin such as meats and dairy products whereas vegans get all their vitamin A from beta-carotene. Beta-carotene is found in certain vegetables and is converted into vitamin A in the body.

Good sources of beta-carotene are carrots, curly kale, red peppers, broccoli, spinach, tomatoes, apricots, cantaloupe, mango and pumpkin.

Cooking actually increases the body's absorption of beta-carotene from the food as does the addition of small amounts of fat to meals. Chopping and puréeing the vegetables may also increase its availability.

recommended daily supplements for your vegan child aged 0–5 years

Breastfed

0–1 month	0.3 ml Abidec Multiviatamin drops
1–12 months	2.5 ml Ketovite liquid and 1 Ketovite tablet
1–2 years	5 ml Ketovite liquid and 1 Ketovite tablet

Bottle-fed

0–2 years taking 500 ml formula daily or more	No vitamin supplement required

Older children

2–5 years	½ tablet VEG 1 or 5 mls Ketovite liquid and 1 Ketovite tablet or another suitable vitamin supplement recommended by GP or dietitian

take special care that vegetarian and vegan diets include sufficient

- Iron
- Zinc
- Omega-3 and omega-6 oils
- Vitamin D
- Protein

Extra care is needed to ensure that vegan diets include:

- Vitamin B_2 (riboflavin)
- Vitamin A
- Vitamin B_{12}
- Iodine
- Calcium

It is important also that the diet provides enough calories for the energy needed by the child.

essential vitamin supplements for vegan breastfed infants

- Vitamin B_{12}
- Vitamin D
- Vitamin B_2 (riboflavin)

Zinc

Zinc is mainly found in foods of animal origin such as meat and fish. Dairy produce also contains zinc so vegetarians have less risk of zinc deficiency than vegans. Zinc deficiency can cause poor immunity, poor wound-healing and taste disturbances. While overt signs of zinc deficiency are rare, you should take care to include sources of zinc in your child's diet.

The absorption of zinc into the body, like iron, can be reduced by phytates. The richest sources of zinc are mainly animal and it is believed that animal protein enhances zinc absorption. Again, as with iron, the body may adjust to a lower level of zinc intake and as a result absorb more from the diet.

Suitable sources of zinc for vegetarians and vegans

- Tofu
- Wholemeal bread
- Fortified breakfast cereals
- Lentils
- Beans
- Chickpeas
- Almonds (ground)
- Smooth nut butter
- Pumpkin and sunflower seeds (ground)

  For vegetarians only
- Dairy products and eggs

Note Whole and chopped nuts are not suitable for children under 5 years of age.

Zinc content of foods suitable for vegetarians and vegans

Food	Zinc mg
2 tablespoons boiled lentils (80 g)	1.1
1 small tin baked beans (200 g)	1.0
Hummus 50 g	0.7
Kidney beans, cooked, 2 heaped tablespoons (70 g)	0.7
Tofu, 60 g, steamed and fried	1.2
1 heaped teaspoon of tahini	1.0
1 slice whole meal bread (35 g)	0.6
Suitable for vegetarians only	
1 glass full fat-milk (200 ml)	0.8
1 ounce cheddar cheese (28 g)	1.2
125 g full-fat yogurt	0.9
1 egg	0.8
Tahini 1 heaped teaspoon	1.0

avoid nuts for children under 5

Whole and chopped nuts are not suitable for children under 5 years due to a risk of choking. Children should never be left unattended when eating nuts.

how to add oil to your child's diet

- Cook with oil
- Drizzle oil onto a salad (walnut oil especially)
- Drizzle olive oil onto crusty bread
- Add oil to pasta dishes (e.g. pasta with olive oil, grated parmesan cheese and chopped tomatoes)

Recommendations for zinc intake

- Children aged 1–3 years need 4 mg zinc a day
- Children aged 4–6 years need 6 mg of zinc a day

How to add calories to your vegetarian or vegan child's diet

Children have high requirements for energy and need to consume a large number of calories relative to their body size. Vegetarian and vegan diets tend to contain a lot of fruits and vegetables which, although they are very nutritious and necessary to the diet, are low in calories. Beans, peas and lentils are very nutritious and high in protein but again are low in calories. This means that a child has to eat quite a lot of these foods to get enough calories from them but since they are also all high in fibre they tend to be 'bulky' and can be very filling, especially for a child. So ways must be found of adding calories to your child's diet. See below for ideas on how to do this.

Add oils to your child's diet

Oils, often portrayed in the media as being bad for your health are very necessary for your vegetarian or vegan child. They are 'energy dense'. This means that a small amount of them can provide lots of calories.

Not only do they provide calories but they also provide polyunsaturated and monunsaturated oils that are good for your child's heart. As we have seen, certain oils such as rapeseed, flaxseed and walnut oils also provide essential fatty acids such as omega-3.

Oils include olive oil, vegetable oil, sunflower oil, olive oil, rapeseed oil, walnut oil. They can be used directly in salad dressings and the like or you can cook with them or they can be consumed in foods such as avocado.

main types of fat provided by different types of oil		
Polyunsaturated oils (omega-6)	Polyunsaturated oils (omega-3)	Monounsaturated oils
Sunflower oil	Flaxseed oil	Olive oil
Corn oil	Walnut oil	Canola oil
Safflower oil	Rapeseed oil	Rapeseed oil
	(also contains monounsaturated fat)	
Cottonseed oil		

Note Most oils contain certain amounts of saturated, monounsaturated and poly-unsaturated fats—the above table refers to the *main* type of fat in the oil.

Add calories with spreads

Spreads are energy-dense and are a useful way to add a few extra calories during the day. Butter and margarines can be used by vegetarians and are high in fat and calories. Although many adults tend to cut back on these foods to help control their weight or their cholesterol levels, there is no need for your child to do this unless overweight.

Spread butter or margarine onto bread, crackers, plain biscuits and potatoes to add extra calories to your child's diet. If you are concerned about the levels of saturated fats in butter, choose a margarine that contains polyunsaturated or monounsaturated oils and use liberally. Avoid low-fat spreads, unless your child is overweight.

Vegan-friendly spreads

There are a number of vegan-friendly spreads available in supermarkets in Ireland. 'Pure' and 'Provamel Bio Soya cook and spread' are two such vegan spreads. You should give them to your child spread on bread, crackers, plain biscuits, potatoes and vegetables to add extra calories.

foods with a high oil content

Suitable for vegetarians and vegans

- **Smooth peanut butter** is a handy sandwich-filler for school and is very nutritious. Other types of nut-spreads are available in health food shops.
- **Tahini** is a spread made from sesame seeds which is high in calories and a good source of iron, zinc and calcium. It can be spread on bread or crackers and is a great sandwich-filler. It is widely available in supermarkets.
- **Hummus,** a spread made with chick-peas, tahini and oil, is high in calories and protein and a good source of iron. Like tahini, it can be spread on bread or crackers and is a great sandwich-filler. It is widely available in supermarkets.
- **'Pure' and 'Provamel Bio Soya** cook and spread' are available in supermarkets.
- **Avocados** are high in oils (especially monounsaturated) and high in calories. They also contain a lot of vitamin E and are delicious in a salad or made into guacamole and used as a dip with tortilla chips.
- **Olives** are an acquired taste for some children but contain lots of monounsaturated oil and are also high in vitamin E.

Suitable for vegetarians only

- **Pesto** is made from olive oil, pine nuts and parmesan cheese and is delicious on pasta, in sandwiches or as a dip. It can be bought in a supermarket or you can make your own. Pesto contains parmesan cheese so is suitable for vegetarians only.

fibre is generally good for health as it keeps the bowel healthy and can help reduce the risk of cardiovascular disease. However, it has little nutritional value so children should not be given too much as it may displace more important nutrients. Children on vegetarian and vegan diets get lots of fibre so there is no need to worry that they are not getting enough. For them it is best to use a combination of wholemeal and white breads throughout the day. Use white pasta and rice more regularly than brown versions.

Soya products for vegan diets

Soya products can provide calories to children on vegan diets as well as protein, calcium and other nutrients. Soya milk is lower in calories than cow's milk. If possible use soya milk that is fortified with calcium, vitamin D and vitamin B_{12}. Soya milk is often sweetened with juices or flavourings to make it more palatable so can contain considerable amounts of sugar. Dental hygiene is even more important than usual if your child is drinking these milks regularly.

Some of the flavoured soya milks can be quite high in calories (up to 85 calories per 100 ml) and may be useful for children who are underweight.

Soya-based desserts, yogurts and cream are also available in Irish supermarkets and again are a useful source of calories for children who are underweight. They also add variety to the diet of a vegan child.

Soya-based cream contains almost as much calories as regular cream and can be added to soups, sauces and desserts.

Dairy products for vegetarians

Dairy products—milk, cheese and yogurt—are the backbone to the diet of vegetarian children and they need a really good intake of dairy products.

Not only do dairy products provide calories and fat, they are also an excellent source of protein, calcium, vitamin B_{12} and vitamin A to the growing child.

Dairy products do contain saturated fat but since a child on a vegetarian diet has no intake of saturated fat from meat sources there is no need to be concerned about its effect on heart disease etc.

In addition, a child's weight gain and growth takes priority over all other dietary factors and if full-fat dairy products are needed to promote this growth, then they are necessary to the well-being of the child and need to be eaten regularly. All vegetarian children should consume at least 3 portions of dairy products a day. However, the average child should not consume more than 600 ml of milk a day in order not to take away the appetite for solid foods.

Recommendations for full-fat, semi-skimmed and skimmed milk
- Children aged 1–2 years should drink full-fat milk.
- Children aged 2–5 years can be offered semi-skimmed milk.
- Children over 5 years can be offered skimmed milk

If you are in any way concerned that your child is underweight, or not eating a varied diet, you should offer full-fat dairy products, otherwise it is fine to offer semi-skimmed or skimmed dairy products as above. The skimmed and semi-skimmed versions contain the same amount of calcium as full-fat milk. If your child is overweight, it is generally best to choose semi-skimmed and skimmed versions of dairy products.

The table below shows the importance of dairy products for a vegetarian child.

nutrients in milk	1 glass (200 ml) full-fat milk	Daily needs of an average 3-year-old
Calories	130.0 kcal	1330.0 kcal
Fat	7.0 g	52.0 g
Protein	6.4 g	15.0 g
Calcium	230.0 mg	800.0 mg
Iron	0.1 mg	8.0 mg
Vitamin A as retinol	60.0 ug	400.0 ug
Vitamin B_{12}	1.8 ug	0.7 ug

My son does not like milk; how can I increase his intake of dairy products?

■ Encourage him to eat cereal in the morning; even non-milk drinkers will generally eat cereal and this will provide at least 100 ml milk. You could also make his porridge with milk instead of water.

■ Add milk into mashed potato.

■ Make smoothies with natural yogurt.

■ Try giving him a hot chocolate, made with hot milk, before bed (remember to brush his teeth afterwards!)

■ Give yogurt as a snack or with stewed fruit as a dessert.

■ Use cheese as a sandwich-filler and add it to omelettes and quiches.

■ Make cheesy dinners such as macaroni cheese or pasta bake with mozzarella cheese

■ Make a cheese sauce for vegetables

■ Grate cheese into mashed potato and pasta dishes

■ If your child's intake of dairy products is especially poor try adding 1 tablespoon of skimmed milk powder to soups or hot drinks for extra protein and calcium.

> **skimmed milk powder** is available in the supermarket under the name 'Marvel'. It contains high biological value protein and is a good source of calcium. If you are concerned about your child's intake of dairy products you could try adding 1 heaped tablespoon to his or her diet everyday. This will provide an extra 5 g protein and 160 mg calcium a day. Do not give your child under 5 any more than 1 heaped tablespoon a day as it is possible to give too much protein! Skimmed milk powder is not suitable for children under 1 year.

Calcium for vegan children

Vegan children can get calcium from a number of sources. One of the main sources for vegans is soya products (milks, yogurts, fortified tofu) that are fortified with calcium so make sure you choose the fortified varieties. Rice and oat milks are also generally fortified with calcium.

Fortified soya, rice and oat milks generally contain about 120 mg calcium per 100 ml. Calcium-enriched orange juices are also now available in Irish supermarkets and generally contain about 120 mg of calcium per 100 ml.

Certain vegetables and fruits also contain calcium. However, some also contain a compound called oxalate that can negatively affect the absorption of calcium from the vegetable. Some green vegetables such as broccoli, kale, okra, bok choy, collard and mustard greens and chinese cabbage have low amounts of oxalate and so the calcium in them is easier for the body to absorb.

Oranges, baked beans, dried figs, almonds, tahini and fortified cereals are also sources of calcium for vegan children. Some cereals are far higher in calcium than others. Ready Brek, for example, contains 400 mg calcium in one bowl before adding milk. 1 tablespoon of black molasses (treacle) can provide as much as 180 mg of calcium. Tofu that is set with calcium is another good source for children.

The Food Safety Authority of Ireland recommends that children aged 1–5 take 800 mg of calcium daily. This is a higher intake than that recommended in the UK.

Calcium content of various foods suitable for vegans

Food and portion size	Calcium content mg
1 glass soya milk (depends on brand)	240
1 soya yogurt (depends on brand)	120
1 glass fortified orange juice	240
1 bowl Ready Brek (30 g)	400
1 tablespoon treacle (molasses)	180
1 orange	75
2 heaped teaspoons tahini (38 g)	260
1 tin baked beans	100
5 dried figs	250

Protein

Proteins are made up of amino acids which are used in the body for different functions. Some amino acids cannot be made by the body and have to be eaten in the diet. These are called essential amino acids.

Proteins that come from meat, fish, dairy products and eggs are all high in essential amino acids and are known as *high biological value* protein. Vegetarians get all their essential amino acids from dairy products and eggs. This is why it is so important that your vegetarian child eats a good supply of dairy products and eggs.

Children on vegan diets generally have no problem eating enough protein. However, protein in plant-based foods such as bread, rice and beans is considered *low biological value* because it doesn't contain all the essential amino acids.

On vegan diets when all the protein comes from plant-based foods certain varieties and combinations need to be eaten to ensure that all of the essential amino acids are eaten.

Instead of getting all the essential amino acids from one food, your child gets them from a combination of foods. This is also known as 'protein complementation' (because the different proteins are complementing each other). Protein complementation is now considered a little old-fashioned by some in the world of nutrition; however, it is no harm to be aware of how to combine proteins to ensure a good balance of amino acids throughout the day (see box above).

protein combinations for vegans

The following combinations of proteins will ensure the diet contains adequate amounts of all the essential amino acids:

- Pulses with rice, for example, rice with dahl, or lentil curry with rice
- Pulses with cereals, for example, beans on toast, falafel with pitta bread
- Nuts with cereals, for example, peanut butter sandwich, nut roast

textured vegetable protein or TVP

is a meat substitute made from soybeans. You can usually find it at your local health food shop.

It is not necessary to consume all the protein combinations at exactly the same time; they can be eaten over the day.

Due to the lower digestibility of plant proteins, children on a vegan diet need to consume more protein than children on vegetarian or meat diets.

good sources of protein for vegetarian and vegan children

- Pulses (beans, peas, lentils and soya products)
- Smooth nut spread
- Seed spread e.g. tahini
- Grains (wheat, rice, oats, pasta, bread, barley etc)
- Tofu

For vegetarians only
- Eggs
- Dairy products
- Quorn
- TVP

Children's daily protein needs:
- Age 1–3 years 15 g   Vegan 15–20 g
- Age 4–6 years 20 g   Vegan 20–25 g

protein content of foods suitable for vegetarians and vegans

Food	Protein per portion
1 slice whole meal bread (35 g)	3.5 g
1 slice white bread	2 g
2 tablespoons cereal (20 g)	2 g (depends on cereal)
1 small tin beans (200 g)	10 g
1 portion tofu, steamed, fried (60 g)	14 g
1 glass soya milk	7 g
1 heaped tablespoon boiled white rice (40g)	1.0
1 tablespoon cooked pasta (30g)	1.0
1 soya yogurt	5.0
Lentils boiled, two tablespoons	6.0
Tofu, 60g	4.6
Peanut butter, 1 tablespoon	3.5
Tahini, 2 heaped teaspoons	7.0
Kidney beans boiled, 2 heaped tablespoons	6.0
Vegetarians only	
1 egg	7.0 g
1 glass milk	7.0 g
1 yogurt (125 g)	7.0 g
1 portion quorn (30 g)	4.0 g
1 portion cheese (30 g)	7.5 g

soya is an effective source of protein

It is interesting to note that soya protein, when evaluated using a method of protein evaluation called PDCAAS (protein digestibility corrected amino acid score), was found to be able to meet protein needs as effectively as animal protein.

treacle

is a thick syrup created from the processing of sugarcane or sugar beet into sugar. In North America it is known as molasses.

Children need 2–3 portions of protein foods per day. Portion size depends on the child's age.

protein foods and portion sizes

Food	Approximate portion size age 1–3 years	Approximate portion size age 3–5 years
TVP	30–60 g	60–90 g
Lentils/beans	1–2 tablespoons	2–3 tablespoons
Tofu, steamed and fried	30–60 g	60 g
Vegetarians only		
Peanut butter	1–2 tablespoons	2 tablespoons
Eggs	½–1 egg	1 egg
Quorn	30–60 g	60–90 g

Quorn (not suitable for vegans)

Quorn is a protein source that serves as a meat-substitute. Products made from it, including quorn mince, quorn chunks and quorn burgers, are found in the freezer section of most supermarkets. It is not suitable for vegans as it contains egg.

The texture of quorn is quite similar to meat and it is generally well-liked and pleasant tasting. It can be used instead of meat in a variety of dishes such as spaghetti bolognese, lasagne, stir-fries, shepherd's pie and many others. It can be given to children aged from 4 months onwards although a baby might not be able to manage the texture until 6 months old.

Quorn is a good source of protein (14 g per 100 g for quorn pieces). It is a high biological value protein providing good levels of all of the essential amino acids. It does not contain any iron. It is not suitable for vegans as it contains egg.

what is quorn?

Quorn is a protein source created by scientists from types of fungus or 'mycoprotein'. It was developed in the 1960s as an alternative source of protein at a time when it was feared there would be food shortages world-wide as populations grew.

Weaning your vegetarian or vegan baby onto solids

The same rules apply for weaning your vegetarian or vegan baby as for all other babies (see Chapter 6). First weaning foods such as puréed fruits, vegetables and baby rice are suitable for a vegetarian/vegan diet anyhow so there is no real difference in stage 1.

Pulses (peas, beans and lentils) are a good source of protein and iron and should be introduced into your vegan or vegetarian baby's diet in stage 2, when your baby is happily taking first foods. If you decide to wean your baby before the age of 6 months, you can give blended pulses at this stage. Remember to cook them well as this makes them easier for your baby to digest and also breaks down certain compounds that may affect the absorption of minerals such as iron. See page 220 for information on cooking with pulses.

Vegetarian babies can be given dairy foods (yogurt and cheese) early in stage 3 as they provide much-needed calories, protein and calcium.

Vegan babies can be given tofu from stage 3 onwards. It is a good source of protein, iron and calcium. Hummus and nut butters can also be given from stage 3 onwards unless there is a family history of food allergy. (See Chapter 13 for more information on food allergies.)

Iron-fortified breakfast cereals can be introduced early in stage 3 and are a good source of iron for your vegan or vegetarian baby. Don't forget to provide your child with fresh fruit or a small amount of a vitamin C containing drink such as diluted fruit juice to aid with iron absorption when taking an iron containing food.

Some commercial baby foods are fortified with vitamins and minerals which can be beneficial for vegan babies, especially vitamin B_2 and B_{12}.

Good iron-sources for vegetarian and vegan babies

- Puréed/mashed beans
- Puréed/mashed lentils
- Fortified breakfast cereals
- Puréed/mashed green vegetables
- Hummus
- Tahini
- Dried fruit
- Tofu

For vegetarians only

- Well-cooked egg

Useful finger foods include chunks of tofu, avocado or rice-cake spread with tahini or smooth peanut butter.

Meal planning for your vegan child

Milk for the vegan child

Most vegan children drink soya milk which can be given from the age of 2 years upwards. Before that it is recommended that vegan children drink soy formula or breast milk as their main drink.

Rice and oat milks are also available and suitable for vegans. However, they tend to be very low in protein and calories and while they contain adequate amounts of calcium if fortified, it may be better to give them to your child as an occasional drink rather than as a staple part of their diet. You can find soya, rice and oat milks in supermarkets in both the shelves and fridge sections.

nuts in vegetarian and vegan diets

Nuts are a useful food as they are high in calories and protein and are very nutritious. If there is no family history of allergies, you can give your child smooth, nut-containing products, for example smooth peanut butter, from stage 2 or 3 of weaning.

Whole and chopped nuts are a choking hazard and should not be given to children less than 5 years old, and children eating nuts should always be supervised.

If your child is at high risk of food allergy (see Chapter 13), you may need to delay introducing nut-containing products until the age of 3 years. In the case of a vegan baby who is at high risk of allergy excluding nuts may cause difficulty obtaining essential nutrients so advice from a dietitian should be obtained.

Try to choose a soya milk that is fortified with calcium and vitamins, particularly vitamin D and vitamin B_{12}. Look out for own-brand supermarket versions as some can be better value for money.

Important energy-dense foods for vegan children:

- Oils
- Vegan spreads (margarines)
- Nuts
- Avocados
- Soya milk, yogurt and desserts
- Tahini and hummus
- Olives
- Soya cream

Recommended daily portions of food types for vegetarian and vegan children

The portion sizes given below are approximate only. The size and number of portions needed will vary depending on your toddler's size, age and activity levels.

Age 1–3 years

- Cereals, breads, potatoes—4 portions a day
  ½–1 slice bread,1–2 tablespoons breakfast cereal, ½–1 Weetabix, ½–1 whole potato, 1–2 tablespoons cooked rice or pasta
- Fruit and vegetables—2–4 portions a day
  ½ apple/pear/ banana, ½–1 plum/kiwi/mandarin, 6 grapes, 4 strawberries, 1 tablespoon tinned fruit, ½ carrot (1 tablespoon), 1 tablespoon cooked vegetables, 2 tablespoons salad vegetables, 2 cherry/½ tomato, 1 small bowl vegetable soup
- Calcium-containing foods—3 portions a day
  200 ml milk (cow/soya/rice), 1 oz (30 g) cheese (vegetarians only), 1 average pot (125 g) yogurt (cow/soya)
- Alternatives to meat—2–3 portions a day
  ½–1 egg, 1–2 tablespoons (30–60 g) TVP/Quorn (vegetarians only), 30–60g Tofu, 1–2 tablespoons beans/lentils, 1–2 tablespoons smooth peanut butter

Age 3–5 years

- Cereals breads, potatoes—4–6 portions a day
  1 small slice bread, 2–3 tablespoons breakfast cereal, 1–1½ Weetabix, 1–1½ whole potato, 2–3 tablespoons cooked rice or pasta
- Fruit and vegetables—2–5 portions a day
  1 small apple/pear/banana, 1 plum, kiwi, mandarin, 8–12 grapes, 6 strawberries, 2 tablespoons tinned fruit, 1 small carrot (2 tablespoons), 2 tablespoons cooked

tips for adding calories to your baby's diet

For vegetarians and vegans
- Add breast milk or formula to puréed foods instead of water
- Serve fruit purées with full-fat natural yogurt or soya yogurt (after 4 months)
- Use olive oil and vegetable oils in cooking
- Add milk/breast milk/formula to soups
- Add milk/breast milk/formula to potatoes
- Give mashed avocado or avocado chunks as a finger food
- Put butter/spread on finger foods such as crackers and plain biscuits
- Put nut butters on finger foods such as crackers and plain biscuits

For vegetarians only
- Add cheese sauce to dinners
- Grate cheese onto mashed potato and pasta

vegetables, 3 tablespoons salad vegetables, 3 cherry/1 small tomato, 1 bowl vegetable soup
- Calcium-containing foods—3 portions a day
  200 ml milk (cow/soya/rice), 1 oz (30 g) (matchbox size) cheese (vegetarians only), 1 average pot (125 g) yogurt (cow/soya)
- Alternatives to meat—2–3 portions a day
  1 egg, 2–3 tablespoons (60–90 g) TVP, 2–3 tablespoons (60–90 g), Quorn (vegetarians only), 60 g tofu, 2–3 tablespoons beans/lentils, 2 tablespoons smooth peanut butter

Cooking pulses (beans, peas, lentils)

Beans, peas and lentils are an excellent source of protein and iron for your baby. Most dried pulses need to be pre-soaked before cooking to allow them to cook better and to get rid of compounds called 'phytates' which can prevent your baby from properly absorbing the iron and other minerals in them. Certain pulses such as yellow split peas and red split lentils do not need to be soaked before cooking.

Soak dried pulses

Place your dried kidney beans, or whatever variety of pulses you are using, in a large bowl and allow to soak either overnight or for 6–8 hours. Allow about 2 pints of water per 450 g of pulses (1 lb). It's a good idea to soak more pulses than you need as they can be kept for several months in a plastic box in the freezer.

Cook the pulses

Before cooking, drain the soaking water and then place the pulses in a saucepan covered in fresh, cold water. Add an unpeeled onion, unpeeled carrot and a bouquet garni for flavour.

Check the cooking information on the packet for how long the pulses need to be boiled. For example, dried kidney beans need to be boiled fast for the first 10 minutes to destroy toxins that are present. Then lower the heat and simmer gently for 45–60 minutes. Dried soya beans need to be boiled vigorously for an hour to destroy the natural toxins contained within the beans. They then need to be simmered for 2–3 hours.

Cook the pulses with the lid of the saucepan on. When cooked, drain the water and discard the vegetables. The cooking water can be kept and used as a stock.

Tinned pulses are already cooked and can be a handy alternative to dried pulses that have to be soaked and cooked. Baked beans are widely used and are an excellent source of protein and iron.

When buying tinned pulses, check the nutritional information to ensure there is not too much added salt or sugar.

Preventing obesity and overweight

15

One in five children and teenagers in Ireland is overweight or obese. Since it is highly likely that obese children will become obese adults this trend has huge implications for the health of the people of Ireland. With so much availability and marketing of junk and fast foods it can be difficult for parents to ensure that their children eat healthy diets. It is vital, however, to establish good eating habits in early life as these habits are likely to last into adulthood. In this chapter we advise you how to help your child to acquire good healthy eating habits.

The National Children's Food Survey carried out in 2005 found that 1 in 5 Irish children is overweight and 1 in 20 is obese. The National Teenagers Food survey carried out in 2007 found that 1 in 5 Irish teenagers is overweight or obese. In 1990 11 per cent of boys and 14 per cent of girls in Ireland were overweight or obese. By 2004 that figure had risen to 20 per cent of boys and 23 per cent of girls. This worrying trend suggests that obesity will be one of the most common and serious nutritional problems in the 21st century.

Causes of obesity

While there are medical causes for obesity, the incidence of such causes is very low (less than 5 per cent). Often parents feel that a child has a natural tendency towards being overweight, maybe because another family member is overweight. However, while genetics (family tendencies) can have an effect on your child's weight, most studies have found it difficult to separate environmental from genetic factors. The fact is, we really don't know how much or how little genetic make-up affects the chances of becoming obese. In our experience, lifestyle and environmental factors are the main contributors to overweight: these are the main causes of overweight in most of the children we see in our outpatient clinics.

Studies have shown that obese children are more likely to have parents who are overweight than children who are not overweight. In 90 per cent of cases one or both parents of an overweight child are also overweight. However, obesity cannot be attributed to genetics alone as children of overweight parents are more than likely to be eating similar foods to their parents and making the same lifestyle choices when it comes to physical activity. Most importantly, the recent rise in obesity rates in Ireland cannot be explained purely on genetic grounds, if at all.

Why worry if your child is overweight?

A child who is overweight is often described as having 'puppy fat'—the parents feel their child will grow out of it. The reality is that children who are overweight are 50 per cent more likely to be overweight as adults and this brings with it associated health risks, including cardiovascular disease, diabetes, high blood pressure and osteoarthritis. Adolescents who are overweight have an 80 per cent chance of being overweight as adults and may already have high blood pressure and raised blood cholesterol levels. Type 2 diabetes, which was previously seen only in older adults and adults who are overweight, is now being detected in obese adolescents. In addition, being overweight as a child can have psychological implications. Overweight and obese children often suffer from impaired social interaction and poor self esteem. Bullying can also be a problem.

Growth and development

As childhood is a time of growth when body weight gradually increases over time, children need a balanced diet, adequate in calories and protein to promote optimal growth and development. Healthy eating policies apply to all children. A parent who is concerned that their child is overweight should see a dietitian before attempting any calorie reductions in the child's diet as it is very important that he or she is not deprived of any vital nutrients such as calcium and iron. In general, we do not recommend that overweight children lose weight, depending on the degree of overweight. We usually encourage overweight children to 'grow into their weight' by attempting to prevent any further weight gain; the child continues to grow taller and eventually reaches the correct balance of height and weight. However, a child who is classed as obese may need to lose a certain amount of weight.

Monitoring progress
If your child is attending a dietitian, she or he will measure your child's weight at each appointment so you can monitor your child's progress. If you are not attending a dietitian and are wondering how frequently to weigh your child, roughly once a month is about right. Too frequent weighing will make your child even more aware of his or her weight and may encourage an unhealthy obsession with the weighing scales.

It is important to be very sensitive about weight and dietary intake where children and adolescents are concerned. Making weight and food an issue can lead to an eating disorder or damage to the child's self-esteem. A family-based approach is the best way to avoid this occurring.

A family-based approach is best

The home is obviously the best place to start when dealing with a child's eating habits. The National Children's Food Survey showed that Irish children aged 5–12 years consume 90 per cent of their daily diet within the family home. This means parents have a huge influence over what their children eat. Irish teenagers consume 75 per cent of their diet at home (National Teens Food Survey, IUNA 2008); this still allows for plenty of parental influence. However, the earlier you introduce your children to good eating habits, the more likely it is that the healthy habits will continue into adult life.

Whether your family consists of two people or 10 people, an excellent way of tackling your child's overweight is by involving everyone in the new 'healthy lifestyle'. Not only is it unfair to prevent your overweight child from eating crisps while allowing brothers and sisters to munch away to their heart's content, it is also counter-productive as your overweight child will feel resentful and unhappy. The same applies to dragging your overweight child out for a walk while the others are allowed to stay at home and watch

Be a good role model

Children's eating habits generally mirror those of their parents so it is hugely important that you are a good role model for your child, eating a healthy diet and getting plenty of exercise. From previous surveys we know that only a fifth of Irish adults eat enough fruit and vegetables every day: how can we expect children to eat 5 portions of fruit and vegetables a day when we adults fail to do so? We also know that parents who are reluctant to try new foods tend to have children who are fussy eaters. So again, if you are trying to encourage your child to try more foods, show that you too are prepared to do so.

television. This scenario may also reinforce feelings of low self esteem and lead your child to believe that exercise and healthy eating are punishments to be endured.

Try putting across the idea that 'it's about time we (the family) all got a bit healthier'. Lifestyle changes and not crash diets are the only way to reach and maintain a healthy weight in the long term. Involve the whole family in walks, trips to the swimming pool or cycle rides. Studies show that habits of activity developed during childhood are commonly maintained into adulthood. Therefore, if you encourage your child to be active, he or she is more likely to be active in later life.

Try to make the following changes in your household:

- Stop buying junk foods—if they aren't in the press, they aren't a temptation
- Leave a large bowl of fruit in a central place in the house for everyone to snack on
- Get rid of the deep fat fryer and use other cooking methods such as steaming, boiling and baking
- Encourage your child to walk or cycle to school (if safe and feasible)
- Start a regular activity such as a Sunday walk or a Saturday morning trip to the swimming pool
- If not doing so already, encourage everyone in the family (including parents) to eat breakfast.

The importance of a balanced diet

Having a healthy body weight depends on the balance between the amount of energy obtained from the food eaten every day and the amount of energy burned off through exercise, activity and growth. It is a simple concept but something people struggle with. If you eat more food than you burn off, you will gain weight. Although children, unlike adults, have an extra energy need for growth, they will still gain excess weight if they eat more than they need.

The types and quantities of foods that your child eats and drinks every day are obviously going to have a major influence on his or her body weight. We know from studies carried out in Ireland such as the National Children's Food survey and the National Teens Food Survey, that diet must be playing a part in the rise of obesity in Ireland. These studies tell us that 40 per cent of children aged 5–12 years and over half of all teenagers are taking too much fat in their diets.

A healthy diet

People often see a healthy diet as some kind of ideal that is extremely difficult to achieve, that unless you are shovelling bran onto your cereal and chewing on chickpeas until your jaws ache you are not eating a healthy diet. It is this idea that a healthy diet is a penance to be done that results in people trying too hard and then being unable to maintain their efforts. A healthy diet is quite simply a diet that contains all or most of the things that the body needs to keep itself in good working order and not too much of the things that aren't so good for it. There is room for chocolate in a healthy diet and there is room for ice-cream in a healthy diet. The key is moderation.

The food pyramid and weight management

The food pyramid is the best model we have of how much of each type of food we should be eating throughout the day. The Department of Health launched the new updated food pyramid in December 2016. The new food pyramid is a healthy eating guide for adults, teenagers and children aged 5 years and over.

Food pyramid Food groups & recommended portions	over 5 years
Group 6, Fizzy drinks, sweets, etc.	**NOT every day**
Group 5, Fats, spreads and oils	eat **in very small amounts**
Group 4, Protein: Meat, chicken, peas, beans, fish, nuts	eat **2 servings** a day
Group 3, Dairy products: Milk, cheese and yogurt	eat **3–5 servings*** a day
Group 2, Starches: Wholemeal bread, cereals, potatoes, rice, pasta	eat **3–5 servings**** a day
Group 1, Fruit & vegetables: Fruit, fruit juice, vegetables	eat **5–7 servings** a day

* Recommended number of servings depends on age: 5 servings for children aged 9–12 years and teenagers aged 12–18 years.
** Up to 7 servings a day for teenage boys and men aged 19–50 years.

Group 1, Fruit & vegetables

Vegetables are generally top of children's most-hated foods list, and fruit tends to be not much further down. This is very unfortunate as fruit and vegetables are low in calories, high in fibre and high in vitamins and minerals. It is recommended that older children eat 5–7 servings of fruit and vegetables a day and younger children (under 5 years) 2–4 servings a day. The National Children's Food Survey found that most Irish children consume just 2 portions a day. The National Teenagers Food Survey (IUNA 2008) found that a third of Irish teenagers consume no fruit at all. It is vital to encourage children to eat fruit early in life so that they will carry this habit into their teenage years and on into adulthood.

At home, have fruit readily available for children. Keep a big fruit bowl in a central location at home where children can pick a piece of fruit on their way out the door or as a healthy snack between meals. Children are always very keen on fruit juices but we do not recommend more than one or two small glasses of fruit juice a day. Fruit smoothies are a good way to encourage eating fruit and can be fun for children to make.

It can require a little more convincing to get your child to eat vegetables. Try offering unfamiliar and more 'exotic' vegetables such as courgettes, mange-tout or sweet potato. If all else fails, your child may take vegetables raw with a dip. See pages 124 and 125 for more ideas on how to increase the amount of fruit and vegetables your child eats.

Fad diets

Diets such as Atkins, South Beach and other 'fad' diets are completely unsuitable for children (and probably for adults too). Not only are they unsuitable but you could damage your child's health irreparably by using them as a means of weight loss/control for your child.

Group 2, Starches

Carbohydrates, from starchy foods like potatoes, pasta, rice and bread, are an important part of our daily diet. The main role of starchy foods is to give us energy. Children should be eating at least 3–5 servings of starchy foods a day, depending on their age and activity levels. Traditionally, foods like pasta and bread have been seen as fattening; however, they actually contain little or no fat: the problem is with the spreads or sauces added to these foods. One slice of bread is about 70–100 calories. One catering-sized pat of butter on that slice adds another 50 calories and a portion of jam adds another 40 calories on top of that. Chocolate spread, a favourite with many children, adds about 110 calories to a slice of bread (and very little goodness despite what the advertisements would lead you to believe!).

The best choice would be a slice of wholemeal bread with a small amount of low-fat spread which adds just an extra 25 calories to the bread.

It is generally better to choose wholemeal varieties of starchy foods for your child aged over 5 years, particularly if he or she is overweight. (Smaller children, less than 5 years old, need less fibre than older children.) Wholemeal varieties contain fibre which passes through the body undigested. This helps regular bowel motions and also fills the stomach which should prevent over-eating. In addition, foods containing wholemeal have more iron and vitamins than white varieties. They also have a lower glycaemic index (see page 234) The gold standard for brown breads is the very high fibre varieties that contain whole-grains. However, if your child will not go for this, you could compromise with something like a multi-grain sliced pan which is particularly useful for sandwiches.

A high-fibre breakfast cereal will also leave your child more satisfied mid-morning and this will help to avoid over-eating at this time. Porridge is high in fibre and will definitely keep your child going. Look at the label on the breakfast cereal and choose one that has more than 6 g of fibre per 100 g of the cereal. However, very high-fibre cereals such as All-Bran are not suitable for young children and adding bran to foods is not recommended for children either. If you are having problems persuading your child to take a high-fibre cereal, you could suggest that they take their high-fibre cereal from Monday to Friday and a different breakfast on Saturdays and Sundays. Alternatively, you could get them to mix a handful of the high-fibre cereal with the preferred cereal every morning.

Group 3, Dairy products

Dairy products provide your child with both protein and calcium as well as vitamins. Children need to maintain a good intake of calcium in order to achieve their optimum peak bone mass, which happens at the end of the teenage years. A child who does not 'bank' enough calcium into the bones before the early 20s, will have a weaker skeleton for the rest of their life. We know that Irish children aren't getting enough calcium in their diets. The National Children's Food Survey showed that 28 per cent of boys and 37 per cent of girls do not get enough calcium in their diets.

In the past, adults may have avoided dairy products with the belief that they are 'fattening', but this is mistaken. Dairy products are not only good for our bones, but also, according to new evidence, they are beneficial in regulating blood pressure and may help control bodyweight. If you choose lower fat varieties, you can avoid the calories and still get the goodness of the protein and calcium. Children and adults need three portions of dairy products a day.

Types of milk
Semi-skimmed milk is also known as low-fat milk and skimmed milk is also known as very low-fat milk.

Children under 2 years of age should be given full-fat milk only. Children over 2 years who are eating well can have semi-skimmed milk and children over 5 years can be given skimmed milk. Fortified low-fat milks are a good choice as they are semi-skimmed, and contain extra calcium and vitamins (e.g. Avonmore Supermilk, Tesco low-fat fortified milk, Dawn Hi-Lo). Don't allow your overweight child to have more than 600 ml milk a day (don't forget to count the milk on breakfast cereal) as it will contribute too many calories to the daily diet overall.

For overweight children over 5 years old it is generally better to choose the low-fat varieties of yogurts. Avoid the much sweetened, high fat yogurts such as Milky Bar, Aero or Rolo yogurts (these are more desserts than yogurts) and the corner-type yogurts with the chocolate crispy parts, except for the occasional treat.

Cheddar cheese is high in fat (about 30 g fat per 100 g) so if your child is overweight it may be best to restrict it to no more than one portion a day. For every block of cheddar that you cut off, remember that a third of it is purely fat. The lower fat varieties still contain a lot of fat (about 20 g per 100 g). Certain cheeses, such as mozzarella and Edam, are naturally lower in fat than Cheddar. Cottage cheese is lower again. Remember that a portion of cheese is about the same size as a matchbox.

Group 4, Protein

Proteins are the building blocks of our bodies and are obviously an important nutrient for children who are growing all the time. The food pyramid advises 2 portions a day to ensure adequate growth. Meat and fish are great sources of protein and also provide your child with important vitamins and minerals. Eggs are another excellent source of protein and can provide a quick and nutritious meal in the form of omelette or scrambled eggs on toast. Beans, peas and lentils are also high in protein and fibre and low in fat and need to be included in particular for children who are vegetarian (see Chapter 14).

Protein-rich foods also tend to be low in fat when unprocessed. Skinless chicken, lean ham, beef, lamb and beans are all low in fat. Unfortunately, however, today's children tend to prefer processed meats and fish. Chicken nuggets, chicken dippers, beef burgers, sausages and novelty hams are all foods that feature regularly in Irish children's diets. The National Teens Food Survey (IUNA 2008) showed that Irish teenagers eat over 50g of processed meats every day: this is far too much. See below for a comparison of fat contents of processed and unprocessed meats:

Fat content of processed and unprocessed meats

Food	Protein per portion	Fat per portion	Calories per portion
Chicken breast (100 g)	32 g	2 g	148
5 chicken nuggets	15 g	10 g	212
Roast beef (90 g)	32 g	5 g	182
2 x frozen burger, grilled, no bun (70 g)	18 g	17 g	230
1 cod fillet, baked (100 g)	21 g	0.7 g	80
3 fish fingers, grilled (84 g)	12 g	7 g	168

If your child is overweight, you need to greatly reduce the amount of these processed foods he or she eats. However, eating chicken nuggets or fish fingers once a week should not cause a problem. If your child will not eat any unprocessed meat then you need to change this eating habit as it may lead to obesity in later life. See Chapter 12 on dealing with food refusal for ways to change your child's attitude to food.

Another important point about protein is that it has a high satiety value—in other words, it 'fills you up'. This is why high-protein diets like Atkins help with weight loss— they prevent the dieter from getting hungry all the time. For example, if you give your child a tuna sandwich for school lunch instead of something like crackers with butter and jam, the tuna is not only more nutritious but it is also far more filling.

Other high-protein and nutritious sandwich fillers include:

- Turkey/chicken
- Boiled egg (avoid mayonnaise)
- Roast beef with mustard
- Lean ham
- Tinned salmon
- Tuna and sweetcorn (no mayonnaise)

Group 5, Fats, spreads and oils

These foods are necessary in the diet, but only in very small amounts. Fats, spreads and oils are a very concentrated source of calories. Always cook with as little fat or oil as possible – grill, oven bake, steam, boil or stir-fry as much as possible. Limit foods containing oil such as mayonnaise, coleslaw and salad dressing. See Chapter 1, pages 4–5, for more detailed information about choosing healthier fats.

Group 6, Fizzy drinks, sweets, etc.

Soft drinks are fine at parties, Christmas etc. but should only be given as a treat and never as part of a child's daily diet.

The top shelf of the food pyramid contains the foods that should be consumed only from time to time and not on a regular basis. These foods include biscuits, confectionery, fried foods, and fizzy drinks. We all know that consuming too much of these foods may cause or contribute to the problem of overweight. Where children are concerned, the best thing to do is to avoid buying these foods completely. Not having chocolate, crisps and biscuits in the house avoids fights.

Fast food

Most children love fast food be it burgers and chips, pizza, or take-away Chinese or Indian. As we all know eating fast food is a very fast way of gaining a few pounds. A 'child's meal' of a cheeseburger, small fries and a small milkshake in a fast food restaurant generally contains over 900 kcal and 30 g fat. A child aged 8 needs about 1850 kcal per day so this meal provides half a day's calories at one sitting.

Visiting a fast food outlet once a week translates into 52 visits a year. This is too many. Try cutting back to once a month at the very most. Why not give your child a different type of treat instead such as visiting the local pool or going bowling?

Treats

Almost all children love treats and there is never a need to completely deny a child a piece of chocolate or a packet of crisps. However, the problem today is that many children are eating 'treats' far too often. According to the National Children's Food Survey 53 per cent of Irish children aged 10–11 years eat sweets every day. This is far too often. Treats are not something children should be given every day.

However, sometimes a child needs a treat, and in this case if your child is overweight bear in mind that some treats are naturally lower in calories than others:

Ice-pops are surprisingly low in calories. If they contain little or no ice-cream they are almost always less than 100 calories. A HB Twister has only 70 calories, and a Loop the Loop contains only 85 calories.

Chocolate Cadbury's Curly-Wurlies, small Dairy Milks and Freddos are lower in calories than other chocolate bars. A Milky Way is also a good choice. Fun-sized bars are also good for treats and generally contain less than 80 calories.

Biscuits The fat and calorie content of various biscuits varies greatly so it is best to check the labels and compare different brands. Jacob's Café Noir are relatively low in fat and calories, as are ginger nuts, fig rolls, jaffa cakes and rich tea biscuits.

Crisps Most crisps are high in fat even if they are advertised as 'low fat'. Popcorn is a healthier alternative to crisps but be sure to buy the ready-to-eat varieties as microwave popcorn can be very high in fat. Tayto Snax are less than 100 calories per bag as are KP Skips and Rancheros. Look out for new rice-based crisps as a lot of these are also very low in fat and calories.

Calories in fruit juice

Pure, unsweetened juices contain the same amount of calories as fizzy drinks. While juices are obviously healthier than these drinks, if your child is drinking a litre of juice a day this adds up to an extra 400 calories. Food and drink companies often market the high vitamin C content of their juices but the reality is that vitamin C cannot be stored in the body. If more is taken than needed the body just pees out the excess. Most juices contain about 30 mg vitamin C per 100 ml. Considering a child needs only 30–40 mg of vitamin C a day, half a glass of juice provides all that is needed without counting the other sources of vitamin C in the diet.

Drinks

While no individual food is alone responsible for the recent increased levels of obesity, soft drinks have definitely had a role in the developing problem of obesity worldwide.

One can of soft drink contains about 130 calories. This is the equivalent of two slices of bread. The problem is that drinking a can of soft drink does not create the same feeling of fullness as eating two slices of bread. In our clinics we have seen overweight children drinking over a litre of soft drink a day (remember a litre is 4–5 glasses). This provides 400 calories a day. A child may only need 1400 calories a day, so this constitutes 30 per cent of their daily energy needs. Most importantly, all these calories come from sugar which will rot the child's teeth. There is absolutely nothing of nutritional value in soft drinks. No protein, no calcium—nothing. Parents should throw out any soft drinks in the house and stop including them in the weekly shop.

Please note also that diet drinks are no more suitable for children than regular soft drinks. They provide absolutely no nutrition and could displace other more nutritious foods from the diet if taken in large quantities.

Children love fruit juice. Advertising suggests that parents are providing their children with great nourishment by giving them juice. However, this is not really the case. The main problem with juices and cordials is that children can rarely stop at one glass. One or two small glasses of juice a day is fine but any more than this can significantly affect your child's total calorie intake.

It is far better for your child to eat the entire fruit than to drink the juice. The entire fruit provides the fibre from the fruit while the juice provides none. The entire fruit is also lower in calories than the juice.

Calorie and sugar content of soft drinks

Drink	Cola etc.	7-Up/Sprite	Apple juice (unsweetened)	Cordial (ready to drink)
Calories per 100 ml	42	43	38	43
Sugar g per 100 ml	10.6 g	11.2 g	9.9 g	10.5 g

As you can see from the table above, all of these drinks are high in sugar and calories. Limit juices and cordials to 1-2 small glasses a day.

So what should I give my child to drink on a daily basis?

All your child should drink on a daily basis is water and milk. If your child is overweight give semi-skimmed or skimmed milk of at most 600 ml a day (approximately one pint). One or two small glasses of juice a day is fine but no more. These could be diluted with water into two or three glasses taken over the day. If your child refuses point blank to drink water, you could flavour it with a dash (only a dash) of sugar-free squash such as Mi Wadi no-added sugar, Ribena Toothkind or an own-brand equivalent.

Snacking

In the past snacking was considered unnecessary and most people survived on '3 square meals' a day. Today, when snacking is the norm, it is often singled out as a trend that may have contributed to the rising obesity problem. However, this is not the case. Studies on children and their snacking habits have found that both overweight children and children with a normal body weight snack. Most dietitians would agree that snacking is a healthy and necessary part of a child's daily diet. The problem generally lies with the type and number of snacks a child eats in a day.

Be very sceptical about claims that certain foods are low in fat or sugar. Read the label and decide for yourself.

A child's diet should be based on 3 meals and 2–3 snacks a day. These snacks should be scheduled at a particular time. Children should not be allowed to wander to the fridge or the cupboard at any time of the day and take whatever they feel like. We refer to this kind of behaviour as 'grazing': the child is getting a continuous stream of food from morning to night, most of which is probably biscuits and juice. A child who is allowed to 'graze' throughout the day may end up eating more food over-all. In addition, the child will probably not have a proper appetite for meals. (An exception to the rule is teenage boys who may graze throughout the entire day and eat all their meals due to their very high energy needs during puberty.)

Good snack times are mid-morning, either in school or at home depending on the age of your child, and again mid-afternoon on return from school. Snacks should be nutritious and just filling enough to help your child to hold out for a few hours before dinner or lunch but without spoiling his or her appetite for the next meal.

Good snack options:
- A fruit or wholemeal scone
- A small bowl of cereal with milk
- A yogurt and a banana (or another piece of fruit)
- Cheese and crackers
- A fruit smoothie made with yogurt
- A bowl of soup with a small bread roll
- A packet of raisins or other type of dried fruit

Always eat breakfast

Twenty per cent of Irish children aged 10–11 years don't eat breakfast on school days. Some parents don't eat breakfast and this is often why children do not. Breakfast is a very important meal for adults and children alike. Breakfast gives children the energy they need to concentrate in school and helps to reduce snacking on sugary foods mid-morning.

If you don't usually eat breakfast try to set an example and sit down for ten minutes in the morning to eat with your child. Even if you just have a banana and a cup of tea that would be a start.

Choose a fibre-rich cereal or porridge for your child for breakfast (see page 226). Cereal creates an opportunity for your child to take some milk also. Some cereals are also fortified with vitamins and minerals that can be beneficial to children. If your child complains of having no appetite in the morning make sure they are not eating late at night before going to bed. If they are still not feeling up to breakfast in the morning, start with something small like a piece of fruit or a yogurt. Eventually your child will start to wake in the morning with an appetite and be hungry for a bowl of cereal or toast.

Portion sizes

So far we have dealt mainly with the types of food your child is eating. More often than not this is the main problem for overweight children. Always start by cutting out junk foods and changing the types of food your child is eating to healthier alternatives. You may be astonished by how easily the quantity of sweets, soft drinks, bars etc. can add up over the day. It may be useful to write down everything your child eats over 2–3 days to get a clear picture of their overall dietary pattern.

If changing the types of food does not help your child to lose weight or slow down weight gain, you will need also to look at how much food they are eating. Although lean meats, fish, pasta, rice and low-fat dairy products are all healthy foods, eating too much of any type of food will provide more calories than the body can burn off resulting in excess weight gain.

It is very important that your child eats slowly and chews food for as long as possible. It can take up to 20 minutes for the brain to register that the stomach is full by which time your child may have totally overeaten. Encourage your child to chew each mouthful entirely and to put his or her fork down several times during the meal to chew.

Serve your child a smaller than normal portion to start with and encourage them to eat slowly. If they have eaten slowly and after 20 minutes still want more, allow a small second portion. It is also a good idea to keep the serving pot on the hob or the work-top, away from the table. If it is sitting on the table, the temptation is to take a second portion before the body has registered that it is full.

Serving meals on smaller plates can help reduce portion sizes without making your child feel as if they are looking at an empty plate.

For more information on portion sizes for younger children see page 127.

Recommended portion sizes at mealtimes for children aged 6–10 years

Starch	Age-appropriate portion size
Cereal	30–40 g
Weetabix	2 Weetabix
Potatoes, mashed	2–3 scoops
Potatoes, boiled	100–150 g
Chips	140 g
Cooked rice	80–120 g (2–3 heaped tablespoons)
Cooked pasta	80–120 g (4–5 tablespoons)
Protein	**Serving size**
Minced meat	90 g
Roast meat	90 g
Fish fillet	90–120 g
Fish fingers/sausages	3*
Pizza	¼ of 9-inch pizza*

* These foods are only to be taken on occasion

Glycaemic index

Glycaemic index (GI) is a very popular concept at the moment. It is a measure of how quickly a food affects the blood sugar and how long the effect lasts before the blood sugar drops again after eating that food. A food with a high GI, for example, a soft drink, will cause the blood sugar to rise very quickly with a subsequent drop. In contrast, foods with a low GI, such as porridge, cause a gradual rise in the blood sugar and sustain them for longer, thus helping you to feel full for longer.

The idea is that by eating foods with a low GI value blood sugars stay stable for longer, thus preventing feelings of hunger and over-eating.

Simple as this may sound, the GI of a food can be affected by a number of other factors such as fat, protein and food structure. For example, ice-cream has a relatively low GI value; however, eating ice-cream is not going to help weight loss, as we all know.

However, GI is worth keeping in mind if your child is overweight. Choose foods that have a low GI but are also low in fat. If you look only at the GI of a food, you may end up choosing foods that have a high fat content which is not going to help your child control their weight. Generally, foods that are higher in fibre tend to have a lower GI.

For example, both Rice Krispies and Weetabix are low in fat; however, Weetabix also has a low GI therefore it is the better choice. Both pears and watermelon are low in fat but pears have a lower GI therefore might make a better snack because they delay hunger.

GI values

Food	GI	Rating*
Baked beans	48	Low
Basmati rice, white	58	Intermediate
Pears	38	Low
Peas	48	Low
Porridge	44	Low
Rice Krispies	82	High
Spaghetti, white	41	low
Spaghetti, wholemeal	37	Low
Watermelon	72	High
Weetabix	69	Intermediate

*High GI—more than 70; intermediate GI— 55–70; low GI– less than 55

Physical activity

Remember that diet really is only one side of the coin—it is so important to encourage your child to be more active in order to maintain a healthy weight and for overall health. A balance has to be achieved between the amount of calories received from food and the amount of calories burned off in physical activity. Without increasing the amount of calories burned off through physical activity, it is very hard to maintain a healthy weight.

One of your main aims when establishing a healthy life style should be to decrease the time your child spends in inactive behaviour (watching TV/playing computer games) as this will ultimately increase the activity.

A lot of overweight children are reluctant to take part in organised physical activity such as sports due to embarrassment at being unfit and general self-consciousness. This does not mean that they cannot be more active. One of the reasons that obesity has increased so much over the last few years is because physical activity within our daily routine has been reduced. We drive to work and school, push a button on a dishwasher instead of washing the dishes and keep our houses very warm so that our bodies do not even need to work to keep warm. If you can get your child more active around the house and as part of their daily routine, you will reduce the need to rely heavily on organised sports and activities to burn calories.

Physical activity can be divided into different categories:

- Activity at school
- Household activity
- Leisure-time activity (playing and sport)

Activity at school is quite hard for parents to influence and unfortunately most schools in Ireland lack the facilities to provide activities that appeal to all children, regardless of weight, age or interests. If your child likes playing sports in school, excellent, but if not there is very little you can do except encourage them to play at lunchtimes outside. Allow your child to walk or cycle to school if it is safe. If the school is too far, encourage public transport if they are old enough, as this generally involves more exercise than being dropped in the car outside the school gates.

Household activity At home, encourage your child to be more active by doing chores around the house such as vacuuming, washing the dishes, washing the car etc.

Involving your child in gardening will also help to increase activity level and it may develop into an interest. If your child is old enough and you have a safe and appropriate mower, allow them to mow the lawn (especially a push-mower).

Watching television

Studies have shown that there is a link between the amount of time spent watching television and obesity. Reducing the amount of time your child spends watching television helps control their weight as they will be forced to do something else which burn more calories (even if it is just complaining!) and may stop them snacking. In fact, it is best not to allow your child to eat while watching television.

Walking the dog is another excellent activity which focuses on the animal rather than the child.

Leisure activities It is good to promote all hobbies your child may develop, even if they are not hugely active, as they will divert attention from snacking and watching TV. If your child is interested in sport already, give lots of encouragement to keep it up. If mainstream sports like soccer, hurling, hockey or basketball do not appeal, suggest skateboarding or BMXing, or dancing or karate. There is a huge range of types of activity, and clubs to join, available to us.

If your child is overweight

- Aim for 3 meals and 2–3 scheduled snacks a day at regular times
- Cut out all soft drinks
- Reduce juices and cordials to 1 glass only a day
- Change to semi-skimmed milk and limit to 600 ml a day
- Aim for 3 servings of low-fat dairy products a day
- Avoid having crisps/chocolate/ice-cream in the house
- Avoid processed meats and foods
- Involve the whole family in a healthy lifestyle
- Reduce the time spent watching TV
- Do not allow snacking while watching TV
- Involve your child in more activity at home

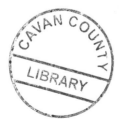

Sources

American Dietetic Association and Dietitians of Canada: position paper 'Vegetarian diets' *J Am Diet Assoc* 2003; **103**:748–65.

Child Growth Foundation *Recommended Growth Monitoring* 2005–6.

ESPGHAN Committee on Nutrition 'Antireflux or Antiregurgitation Milk Products for Infant and Young Children—Commentary' *J Paediatr Gastroenterol Nutr* 2002; **34** (5) 496–8

ESPGHAN Committee on Nutrition 'Complementary Feeding—Medical Position Paper' *J Paediatr Gastroenterol Nutr* 2008; **46** 99–110

ESPGHAN Committee on Nutrition. 'Soy Protein Infant Formulae and Follow-On Formulae—Medical Position Paper' *J Paediatr Gastroenterol Nutr* 2006; **42** 352–61

ESPGHAN Working Group on Acute Diarrhoea 'Recommendations for Feeding in Childhood Gastroenteritis—Guidelines' *J Paediatr Gastroenterol Nutr* 1997; **24**(5):619–20

Food Safety Authority of Ireland 'Information Relevant to the Development of Guidance Material for the Safe Feeding of Reconstituted Powdered Infant Formula' *Guidance Note* 22, 2007

Food Safety Authority of Ireland 'Recommendations for a National Policy on Vitamin D Supplementation for Infants in Ireland' 2007

Food Safety Authority of Ireland 'Best Practice for Infant Feeding in Ireland' 2012

Food Standards Agency (2002) *McCance and Widdowson's The Composition of Foods* Sixth summary edition. Cambridge: Royal Society of Chemistry

Freeman VE, Mulder J, Van't Hof MA, Hoey HMV, Gibney MJ 'A longitudinal study of iron status in children at 12, 24 and 36 months' *Public Health Nutrition* 1998; **1(2)**:93–100.

Gideon Koren. 'Motherisk Update: Drinking Alcohol while breastfeeding' *Canadian Family Physician* 2002 **Vol 48**: 39–41

Hoekstra JH. 'Toddler Diarrhoea: more a nutritional disorder than a disease' *Arch Dis Child* 1998; **79** 2–5

Irish Universities Nutrition Alliance *National Children's Food Survey* 2005 (www.iuna.net)

Irish Universities Nutrition Alliance *National Teenagers' Food Survey* 2008 (www.iuna.net)

NASPGHAN Nutrition Report Committee 'Clinical Efficacy of Probiotics: Review of the evidence with focus on children' *J Paediatr Gastroenterol Nutr* 2006; **43**: 550–7

NASPGHAN 'Evaluation and Treatment of Constipation in Infants and Children – Clinical Practice Guideline' *J Paediatr Gastroenterol Nutr* 2006; **43**: e1–e13

NASPGHAN 'Pediatric GE Reflux—Clinical Practice Guidelines. *J Paediatr Gastroenterol Nutr* 2001; **32**: S1—S29

Nawoor Z, Burns R, Smith DF, Sheehan S, O' Herlihy C, Smyth PPA. 'Iodine intake in pregnancy in Ireland—A cause for concern?' *Irish Journal Medical Science* 2006; **175(2)**: 21–24

Perinatal Lipid Intake Working Group 'Dietary fat intakes for pregnant and lactating women—Consensus Statement' *British Journal of Nutrition* 2007; 98**(5)**: 873–7

Rublin G, Anne D. 'Chronic constipation in children' *BMJ* 2006; **333**:1051–5

Stanley Ip, Mei Chung et al 'Breastfeeding and Maternal and Infant Health Outcomes in Developed Countries' *Evidence Report/Technology Assessment* 2007 Number 153

Glossary

Absorption	In the context of nutrition absorption generally refers to food components (amino acids, glucose, vitamins) travelling across the lining of the gut into the bloodstream.
Agrochemical residues	Traces left on foods from chemicals (mainly pesticides) that are added as part of the farming process.
Alpha-linoleic acid	An essential omega-3 polyunsaturated fat found in a number of oils such as flaxseed, walnut, soyabean, rapeseed and linseed. It is also found in the nuts or seeds themselves (e.g. walnuts). Two important derivatives of alpha-linoleic acid are DHA and EPA.
Anaemia	A condition whereby the red blood cells in the body are either low in haemoglobin or low in number or both. Anaemia can be caused by blood loss, for example during an operation, in which case a person may need a blood transfusion. It can also happen slowly over time from iron deficiency. Either way, as a result the blood is unable to carry enough oxygen around the body. Iron-deficiency is a condition whereby the red blood cells are low in haemoglobin due to a lack of iron in the diet. Pernicious anaemia is type of anaemia caused by an inadequate amount of vitamin B_{12}. Vitamin B_{12} is needed for red blood cell production
Antioxidant	A substance that detoxifies or mops up free radicals (byproducts of chemical reactions of the body or in the environment)
Arachadonic acid (AA)	A type of long chain polyunsaturated fat (omega-6), found in meat. Arachidonic acid is a major component in the structure of the body's cells especially brain, eye and nerve tissue. It has an important role in brain development in foetal and early life. Derivatives of arachidonic acid play key roles in the body's inflammatory response.
Artificial sweetener	An intensely sweet chemical, with minimal calories relative to sugar. Common examples include aspartame, sorbitol and saccharin.
Atopic diseases	Allergic diseases including asthma, eczema, hay fever and food allergy. These diseases have a strong hereditary component. Apart from food there are many different allergens that may provoke symptoms e.g. pollens, house dust mites, pets and mould spores.
Autistic spectrum	A variety of conditions which cause significant impairment of a child's ability to relate to people including parents.
Bilirubin	A normal pigment made when red blood cells break down in the body. It is usually processed by the liver and eliminated in the stool.

Cardiovascular disease	The cardiovascular system is the heart and blood vessels in the body. Cardiovascular disease refers to any disease affecting these vessels. Atherosclerosis, or hardening of the arteries, is one of the main causes of cardiovascular disease.
Chronic	Continuing for a long period of time.
DHA	Docosahexaenoic acid. An omega-3 fat found in oily fish. It can be made in the body from alpha linoleic acid (although, perhaps not very efficiently). DHA has an important role in brain development in foetal and early life. It may also have an anti-inflammatory effect in the body and make the blood less likely to clot.
Eczema	A common skin disorder of infancy and childhood. It is an inflammatory condition that makes the skin itchy. In mild cases the skin is dry and scaly but in more severe cases the skin can be red, blistered and weepy.
Enzymes	A group of complex proteins that play key roles in many biological processes in the body e.g. digestion and metabolism.
EPA	Eicosapentaenoic acid. An omega-3 fat found in oily fish. It can also be made in the body from alpha linoleic acid (although possibly not very efficiently). This type of fat is associated with protection against heart disease as it makes the blood less likely to clot. It may also have an anti-inflammatory effect. Research shows that it may also have a role in helping children with autistic spectrum disorders although more studies are needed.
ESPGHAN	European Society of Paediatric Gastroenterology, Hepatology and Nutrition. This is an international scientific society based in Europe. It is composed of a group of experts in medicine and nutrition who meet regularly and give various recommendations based on the most up to date medical evidence.
Fortified	Where something is added to something else to improve it. For example, a breakfast cereal might be fortified with vitamin C or a milk might be fortified with extra calcium.
Full blood count	A type of blood test where a sample of blood is taken from a person and 'mixed' in such a way that the different types of cells separate out and can be counted or quantified. A full blood count generally gives information on red blood cells, white cells and platelets. It can also give information on how much haemoglobin is in the red cells and on the size and colour of the red cells.
Galactosemia	A life threatening condition where the body is not able to process (metabolise) the sugar galactose. Galactose is part of lactose, the naturally occurring sugar in milk. Early diagnosis and treatment of galactosemia is vital. A life-long lactose-free diet is necessary.

Gluten	A protein in wheat, barley, rye and oats.
Haemoglobin	A protein found in red blood cells that contains iron and carries oxygen around the body. It gives blood its red colour.
Hypoglycaemia	Sugar levels in the blood stream are strictly regulated to keep them within a certain range. Hypoglycaemia occurs when blood sugar levels drop too far. Sugar levels may drop to too low a level if, for example, a baby has had to fast for a long time.
Hypothyroidism	A condition whereby the thyroid gland is not secreting enough thyroid hormone (thyroxine). 'Thyroxine' is a hormone that controls a number of factors in the body including metabolic rate, causing people with hypothyroidism to gain weight more easily. The thyroid gland relies on having enough iodine in the diet to produce adequate levels of hormones. However, there are many reasons why a person may have an under-active thyroid, not necessarily related to iodine.
Immunoglobulin E (IgE)	A specific type of immunoglobulin linked with allergies. It is normally present at very low levels in the plasma. In children or adults with food allergies or other allergic diseases, such as asthma or eczema, levels may be raised.
Immunoglobulins	A whole range of immunoglobulins are produced by the immune system. More commonly known as antibodies, they are important for fighting off infection.
Jaundice	Babies become jaundiced when they have too much bilirubin in their blood. It is quite common in newborns and usually settles once feeding has been established.
Leavening	This takes place when something is added to a dough or a batter (such as yeast) to create bubbles that trap gas (usually carbon dioxide) to produce a 'spongy' effect in a cake or bread.
Linoleic acid	An essential omega-6 polyunsaturated fat found in oils such as sunflower, safflower, corn, canola and soya among others. It is also found in nuts, eggs and lean meat. An important derivative of linoleic acid is arachadonic acid (AA)
Macrobiotic diet	A diet/way of life developed by a Japanese man called George Ohsawa. It is mainly vegetarian in nature although fish is generally allowed. Meat, poultry and dairy products are normally avoided. It is a high-fibre, low-fat diet with a strong emphasis on whole grains, beans, vegetable and soya products. It is quite similar to a vegan diet. Macrobiotic diets are not recommended for children (ESPAGHN 2008).
Maltodextrin	Made from starch and used as a food additive. During digestion maltodextrin is broken down to release glucose. It is easily digested.

Metabolism	The chemical processes that occur in living organisms resulting in growth, production of energy and elimination of waste.
Methylmalonic acid (MMA)	A type of test done sometimes by doctors to help decide if a person is vitamin B_{12} deficient or not. It can also be done for other reasons. An elevated MMA test may indicate a B_{12} deficiency.
Nervous system	Specific parts of the body including the brain, spinal cord and nerves. The nervous system is made up of special types of cells called neurons which transmit electrical impulses allowing reactions to the environment, muscle movement, memory, learning and many other abilities.
Oesophagus	More commonly known as the food pipe. It is a tube connecting the mouth with the stomach.
Oligosaccharides	Carbohydrates made up of small chains (3-10) of simple sugars such as glucose, galactose or fructose. Prebiotics are oligosaccharides.
Omega-3	type of polyunsaturated fat. Alpha linoleic acid is an omega-3 fat. DHA and EPA, found in oily fish are also types of omega-3 fats.
Omega-6	A type of polyunsaturated fat. Linoleic acid is an omega-6 fat. Arachadonic acid (AA) is also a type of omega-6 fat.
Oxalate	Chemical compounds contained in certain plants (including fruits and vegetables). They can bind to calcium, iron and other minerals and prevent them from being absorbed into the body.
Pollens	Fine powders produced by flowers to fertilise other flowers of the same species.
Wheeze	An abnormal sound heard during exhalation. It can be produced by partial obstruction of the lower airway in the lungs. Wheezes may be harsh and low pitched or high-pitched and almost musical.

Index

Index